An Ideological Analysis of Breastfeeding in Contemporary America

An Ideological Analysis of Breastfeeding in Contemporary America

Disciplining the Maternal Body

Loreen N. Olson and Jenni M. Simon

LEXINGTON BOOKS
Lanham • Boulder • New York • London

Published by Lexington Books
An imprint of The Rowman & Littlefield Publishing Group, Inc.
4501 Forbes Boulevard, Suite 200, Lanham, Maryland 20706
www.rowman.com

6 Tinworth Street, London SE11 5AL

British Library Cataloguing in Publication Information Available

Library of Congress Cataloging-in-Publication Data Available

ISBN 978-1-4985-3129-0 (cloth)
ISBN 978-1-4985-3130-6 (electronic)

Contents

Acknowledgments

To Kenyon, Keaton, Keenan, and Reece . . .
we hope we made you proud.

And to Mark and Danny . . .
thank you for giving us the space to mother in our unique ways.
This was your struggle, too—the book, the breastfeeding,
and the bottle feeding!
Thank you for supporting us.

ONE

Discourse, Ideology, and Breastfeeding

The Breast-is-Best Discursive Formation and the Construction of Hegemonic Mothering

In today's society, expecting parents prepare for the baby's arrival by doing all of the pre-planning possible. They are painting the baby's room in some gender-neutral color, buying a 4-in-1 convertible crib, deciding if they really need that heated baby wipe dispenser, stocking up on diapers, weighing the pros and cons of different types of car seats, and, if they don't yet know the sex of the baby, purchasing yellow and green onesies.

In addition to dealing with the stress of checking items off their shopping list, soon-to-be parents are also faced with many tough decisions: to ascribe to the family-bed philosophy or to use cloth or disposable diapers. If they are considering cloth diapers, then they also need to consider the pros and cons of using a laundry service or washing them at home. Bringing a baby home is heady work and not something new parents want to mess up. Even the most mundane decision can seem overwhelming. Yet, if the mother is carrying the baby, she (and her partner) may also be faced with one of the biggest decisions of all: to buy bottles or a breast pump. Said another way, the soon-to-be parents need to decide if the mother is going to breastfeed or formula feed. Importantly, she shouldn't articulate that uncertainty too loudly!

Unbeknownst to them, these soon-to-be parents are in the midst of a dominant "breast-is-best" (Sears, Sears, Sears, & Sears, 2003, p. 117) rhetorical era espoused by many. The message is clear: to be a good parent, one must provide breast milk to the infant for the baby to grow into a healthy, productive citizen. Or, as a character states in Carol Shields'

Pulitzer Prize winning book, *Stone Diaries*, a mother's life isn't worth a plate of cabbage nor does she understand true love if she doesn't breastfeed. Any woman who deviates from this social norm will experience public chastisement from medical professionals, authors of popular press parenting books, relatives, and even strangers in the mall. People have no problem disciplining you for not being the good mother that you should be and declaring you selfish and unconcerned for your child's well-being if you are not breastfeeding your baby. Annie Ferguson Muscato is one such mom who was scolded by a stranger in Target for buying baby formula (Willetts, n.d.). In response, Annie took to social media, posting an open letter to the stranger on her Facebook page. In this letter, she describes her agonizing experience with breastfeeding and how she came to be at peace with formula feeding her child. To follow are excerpts from her post.

> Dear Stranger in Target,
>
> You didn't need to tell me, "breast is best" as I was buying a can of baby formula, because I already know. . . . I know that my husband and I excitedly took the four hour breast feeding class when I was pregnant. . . . I know that we struggled at first. That some nights we both cried together. . . . I know "breast is best" just like you do. . . . But, let me tell you what else I know. I know that my baby began screaming after she ate. Writhing in pain. Inconsolable. . . . And then finally, we tried the hypoallergenic dairy protein free formula you saw me buying today. And the screaming lessened. And my baby started smiling. She started interacting. She started sleeping. And I cried. Because I thought breast was best. I thought my body failed her. . . . I know you think I must not care or I'm lazy, or maybe you were genuinely trying to be helpful and thought no one had ever told me the benefits of breast feeding.
>
> But, you are wrong. What I know that you don't is that breast ISN'T always best. I know happy, healthy baby is best. I know FED is best. . . . So, dear stranger, next time you see someone buying formula, try to remember that mamas should support each other. Think about everything you might not know. Remind yourself that "fed is best" and smile because it means someone loves their baby enough to do what's best for them.
>
> Love, Another Mom Doing Her Best and a Happier Formula Fed Baby

At the time we are writing this book, Annie's post dating back approximately two years has 154,000 likes, 94,000 shares, 25,000 comments. Clearly, Annie's post struck a nerve! As intimated in the post and by others, breastfeeding indeed is one of the ultimate maternal performances that rises to symphonic pitches. In one bodied experience, we see the enactment of the material, maternal, feminist, gendered, sexed, and sexualized. However, the expectations of this maternal act have changed over time. During the eighteenth century, women who were pregnant were encouraged to breastfeed as a "national duty" (Yeo, 2005, p. 7). Conversely, by the middle of the twentieth century, women who wanted to breastfeed were often dissuaded from doing so by formula manufacturers and medical authorities promoting bottle feeding and by social mores equating nursing with eroticism (Koerber, 2006). Thus, the personal decision to breastfeed during this time was often made in defiance of the dominant discourse. However, this norm changed during the latter part of twentieth century. Breastfeeding has once again become the preferred method of infant feeding and pro-breastfeeding the dominant discourse.

Granted, breast milk may provide some benefits over formula, but the latter also provides essential nourishment. In fact, Kramer and colleagues (2008) completed the "largest randomized trial ever conducted in the area of human lactation" and "found no evidence of risks or benefits of prolonged and exclusive breastfeeding for child and maternal behavior" (p. 435). In her book, *Is Breast Best? Taking on the Breastfeeding Experts and the New High Stakes of Motherhood*, Joan Wolf (2011) provides a critical analysis of the epidemiological research which has claimed that breastfeeding provides significant advantages over formula feeding in developed countries. She argues instead that, while breastfeeding appears to modestly reduce babies' gastrointestinal infections, the evidence related to all of the other benefits allegedly associated with breastfeeding is "plagued by selection bias, unexamined confounding variables, and inconsistent outcomes" (Wolf, 2013, p. 307). Moreover, the United States' Surgeon General's Call to Action to Support Breastfeeding (United States, 2011) noted that, after conducting a systematic review of the literature on breastfeeding and maternal and infant health, the Agency for Healthcare Research and Quality's (AHRQ) report

> cautioned that, although a history of breastfeeding is associated with a reduced risk of many diseases in infants and mothers, almost all of the data in the AHRQ review were gathered from observational studies. Therefore, the associates described in the report do not necessarily represent causality. Another limitation of the systematic review was the wide variation in quality among the body of evidence across health outcomes. (p. 2)

Thus, despite the lack of scientific rigor, absence of cause-and-effect relationships, and variable findings, many parents, care providers, researchers, governments, institutions, and the public-at-large still believe that the breast-is-best approach is the only way to properly care for babies. This pro-breastfeeding rhetoric is espoused in books for new mothers and by the supportive, yet authoritative voices of organizations that attempt to dissuade women from giving their babies formula or solid food during the first year (Kotler, 2006). The master narrative (i.e., the most central and dominant social ideology or worldview) perpetuated in these discourses informs mothers that breastfeeding signifies good and proper parenting and should be encouraged above all other forms of feeding for babies to grow into healthy, productive citizens of the society. Such an ideological stance furthers several contemporary feminist critiques of what motherhood has become in U.S. society. For example, *intensive mothering*, identified by sociologist Sharon Hays (1996), "requires not only large quantities of money but also professional-level skills and copious amounts of physical, moral, mental, and emotional energy on the part of the individual mother" (p. 4). Similarily, Douglas and Michaels' (2004) *new mommism* "is a set of ideals, norms, and practices . . . that seem on the surface to celebrate motherhood, but which in reality promulgate standards of perfection that are beyond our reach" (pp. 4–5). Likewise, *total motherhood*, as articulated by Wolf (2013), instructs mothers "to give themselves over completely to eliminating risk and maximizing opportunity for their offspring and that no risk is too small for a mother to ignore and no price too steep for her to bear in the process" (p. 307). The prevailing breast-is-best dogmatism is just one additional way that these maternal performances, no matter the label, create a culture wherein mothers are expected to subordinate their own needs to those of their child's and to do so no matter the economic cost to her and her family.

This current paradigmatic era finds countless women who struggle with or choose not to breastfeed. Now, it is these women who appear to be the ones resisting the dominant discourse surrounding the breastfeeding master narrative. As a result, many of their voices are left out of the parenting books, ostracized in many pre-natal classes, criticized by medical professionals and family members alike, and thereby are made to feel, in part, "left out" of mothering. This book is dedicated to such moms, who, like us, feel left out and less than adequate maternal figures by making the very personal and reasoned decision to formula feed our babies.

Unfortunately, we're not alone. The sheer number of expecting parents who are negotiating life in the midst of this breast-is-best paradigm is cause enough to be concerned about the impact of the ideology. The Center for Disease Control's 2015 statistics (Center for Disease Control, 2018) show that approximately 83 percent of the 3,978,497 children born in the United States were breastfed at birth. But those numbers change dramatically once babies leave the hospital. For instance, babies who had *any* breastmilk drops to approximately 58 percent at six months of age and to 36 percent at 12 months. Conversing this story, these numbers are telling us that 17 percent, 42 percent, and 74 percent of babies are receiving *some* formula at birth, at six months, and at 12 months, respectively. Moreover, less than half (47 percent) are exclusively breastfed for six months and only approximately 25 percent at 12 months.

When you consider that close to 4,000,000 babies were born in the United States in 2015, these numbers reveal that a high percentage and millions of babies are receiving formula in their first year of life. The statistics also indicate that a significantly large number of women are experiencing a very different notion of mothering from the one socially propped up as *THE best way to be a mother*. This book is an attempt to give voice and legitimacy to these women's experiences. It is a feminist oppositional story, a resistance narrative, or a way of talking back. More specifically, the purpose of this book is to unpack the ideology embedded in the U.S. breastfeeding social, political, medical, and institutional discourses from the 1940s and 1950s to today and illuminate how they are working to perpetuate heterosexist, patriarchal viewpoints and to marginalize the voices of women who, for a variety of reasons, do not breastfeed. Specifically, we will explore various governmental, institutional, medical, popular press, and mediated texts directed at new mothers to understand the construction of breast-is-best discourse and how it constrains women's choices and silences their voices. We will also hear first-person accounts about the experiences of what it means to be a mother who bottle fed her child as well as some mediated resistance messages by moms who have taken to the blogosphere to "talk back" to a society that is attempting to assert social control over their bodies and who are "taking back" what it means to be a good mother.

In many ways, this book is *our* way of talking back as a means of taking back our own maternal identities. We too decided at various points and for different reasons to formula feed our babies. We both have two children—Jenni: two boys; Loreen: boy/girl twins. Although the two of us are more than a decade apart in age, our children are similar in age, meaning we lived through the breast-is-best era at approximately the same time. It's fair to say that we both felt some degree of guilt as a result of the decision to formula feed. But, as we reflected upon that guilt and questioned its legitimacy, our internal feminist, social critic voices kicked in, helping drown out the impact of the patriarchal ideology embedded in the pro-breastfeeding discourse and the notions of total motherhood or intensive mothering. We are unapologetic feminists, and this book is unabashedly a feminist critique of that patriarchal control. As cisgendered, white, able-bodied, heterosexual feminist women, we also recognize our own privileged positionality toward this topic—one that is usually the norm by which good, natural motherhood is defined. On one hand, we recognize and honor the fact that breastfeeding is a very feminine act and therefore quite empowering. As noted by Dr. Christine Northrup (2010),

> Countless women have regained trust in their bodies through nursing their children, even if they weren't sure at first that they could do it. It is an act of female power, and I think of it as feminism in its purest form. (p. 516)

Breastfeeding IS an act of female power, for who else can sustain another living human? Believing that we are providing the gift of life is awe-inspiring, spiritual, and humbling—all at the same time. The current pro-breastfeeding movement in the United States is deeply indebted to countless feminist individuals and female friendly groups and organizations. La Leche League International, for example, is a women's organization that "grew from a local, to a national, and then an international organization that has been helping thousands of mothers and babies all over the world for more than 60 years," and is perhaps the most active pro-breastfeeding organization in the United States (LLLI, History). Individuals, like Senator Ted Kennedy, also fostered the pro-breastfeeding movement by orchestrating laws and regulations in the wake of underhanded marketing practices conducted by formula companies. In 1978, Kennedy was chairman of the Senate Sub-Committee on Health and Scientific Research. Following reports that children in developing countries were sick and dying as a result of formula feeding, Kennedy called a Senate hearing in May of 1978 to discuss "the promotion and use of infant formula in developing countries" (Brady, 2012). His hardline questions, like "Can a product which requires clean water, good sanitation, adequate family income and a literate parent to follow printed instructions be properly and safely used in areas where water is contaminated, sewage runs in the streets, poverty is severe and illiteracy high?" (as cited in Brady, 2012), forced the medical community, parents, and lawmakers to rethink their positions on formulated milk.

Yet, similar to how Douglas and Michaels (2004) describe the new momism as inherently contradictory, so too is the pro-breastfeeding movement something that "draws from and repudiates feminism" (p. 5). The act of breastfeeding is both empowering and disempowering for women. It is rather paradoxical that many women may feel empowered by the ability to breastfeed their children, yet, ironically, feel disempowered when something or someone other than themselves is telling them that this is what they need to do in order to be good mothers. The ideological forces of the pro-breastfeeding discourse may also marginalize, and thereby disempower, some women who choose not to or cannot breastfeed their children. Both states can and do co-exist. However, the impact of the current social discourse tends to create false dichotomies—bottle feed *or* breastfeed—forcing women to be either a good mommy (breastfeed) or a bad mommy (bottle feed). It is the duality of the breast-is-best's (dis)empowering nature that forms the nexus of our critique. Our current breastfeeding discourses also reveal a traditional, eurocentric, able-bodied, and heteronormative narrative view of mothering, parenting, and family life. Absent from these narratives are the experiences, of mothers of color (Hill Collins, 2007), LGTBQ+ parents (e.g., Rosswood, 2016), differently abled mothers (e.g., Thomas, 2007), as well as foster and adoptive parents (e.g., Crook, 2017).

As this breast-is-best movement has become more entrenched in medical, [quasi]governmental, institutional, and social hierarchies which misrepresent the benefits of breastfeeding and the risks of formula feeding (Wolf, 2011; 2013), its associated discourses have become a vice grip, squeezing choice and autonomy away from women. These discourses reinforce the ideals of total motherhood (Wolf, 2011; 2013) by telling women what they "should" be doing. Control and choice have been taken away from mothers and placed in the hands of society that has positioned itself to know what is best for women when it comes to having and raising a healthy child. As such, we will argue throughout this book that ascribing to pro-breastfeeding ideologies can lead to a form of hegemonic mothering—wherein good mothers are expected to subvert their own needs, in general, as they elevate their children's. Importantly, they must also submit their bodies and their breasts to these same children as well as to the state. They and their dismembered breasts become the objects of the various intertwining discourses and are to be monitored and punished when not sacrificing everything to provide breast milk to their baby.

It just becomes "common sense" for women and their families to believe in this paradigm and to comply with the breast-is-best mandate. Yet, we assert that one of the most insidious features of power and ideology in language, in general, and in the breast-is-best discourse, more specifically, is the way in which the notion of common-sense has become embedded within said discourse. In fact, it is when particular philosophies or viewpoints become taken-for-granted beliefs and assumptions about the world—or common sense—that their corresponding ideology becomes most effective. Fairclough (1989) calls this "ideological common sense"—a common sense that serves to sustain unequal power relations. There can be no doubt that the breast-is-best perspective has become the common sensical way of performing motherhood post-partum. As such, we argue that this now accepted as the-way-it-is belief about breastfeeding is serving as ideological common sense. As we will demonstrate throughout the book, following this common sense, for example, privileges mothers who do breastfeed, supports the profit making of the motherhood/parenting book writing genre, and helps employ lactation consultants at "baby-friendly hospitals." Conversely, those acting "without common sense," such as mothers who don't breastfeed for whatever reason, or researchers like Joan Wolf (2011; 2013) who offer careful, informed critiques of the science of breastfeeding, or moms like, Annie Ferguson Muscoto who gave her baby formula are chastised, ridiculed, and in some cases shamed in Target for buying baby formula.

Additionally, there is a very dangerous discursive pattern that is associated with ideological common sense—a rhetorical force that easily transports that which is common sensical to that which is natural (Fairclough, 1989). The reason we consider this pattern "dangerous" is because, as discourse is naturalized and turned into common sense, it *appears* to lose its ideological nature and to be "neutral in struggles for power" (Fairclough, 1989, p. 92). Accordingly, individuals operating within the confines of a dominant discourse type (e.g., breast-is-best) just need to learn the skills necessary (breastfeeding techniques) for successfully accomplishing the goals of the discourse and related social hierarchies and institutions, for it is the "natural thing" to do. For example, breastfeeding is a natural act, and mothers just need to develop the skills necessary to properly execute the act of feeding their infant. How much more common sense can there be?

In this type of natural, common sense discourse, which we label the heuristic of the natural, we see that accepting the naturalization of discourse is synonymous with the "emptying of its ideological content" (p. 92). Yet, as noted by Fairclough, this is paradoxical in that "ideology works through disguising its nature, pretending to be what it isn't" (p. 92). Ideology is STILL at work in the naturalization of pro-breastfeeding discourse types and working very hard to discipline mothers into compliance.

As the discourses become naturalized, it is a logical next step that they then become god-given and all related behaviors judged god-like and morally superior. We see such ideology within the development of the contemporary breastfeeding ideology. Breastfeeding is natural, unambiguous, morally superior, and holy. As a morally superior, godly act, it becomes a practice about which to proselytize. Evangelists are everywhere spreading the gospel of the breast! To understand more fully how we have arrived at such a point in time, allow us to step back for a moment and explain the theoretical perspectives that frame our work.

TEXTS, DISCOURSE, POWER, AND KNOWLEDGE: OUR THEORETICAL APPROACH

First and foremost, this work is an archaeological dig into how knowledge and power about the breast-is-best ideology has been discursively formed (Foucault, 2010a; 2010b) in the United States mid-twentieth century to today. Therefore, discourse, or as Foucault asserts, is "thought made visible through words" (Shoshana, 2014) is central in this excavation. Foucault (1990) reminds us that

> *It is discourse that power and knowledge are joined together (emphasis added).* And for this very reason, we must conceive discourse as a series of discontinuous segments whose tactical function is never uniform nor stable. But, to be more precise, we must not imagine a world of discourse, divided by accepted discourse and excluded discourse, or between the dominant discourse and the dominated one; but as a multi-

> plicity of discursive elements that can come into play in various strategies. (Foucault, 1990, p. 100)

This general perspective on discourse allows us to explore the relationships between language, power, and knowledge as related to the breast-is-best paradigm. More specifically, we argue that because of the way disparate pro-breastfeeding discourses relate to one another a discursive formation is created. In their most basic form, discursive formations are composed of language, social structure, and human agency (Foucault, 1994). Discursive analysis examines the relationships between the three, and, in particular, how language shapes social structures and knowledge for the purpose of policing human agency (Foucault, 1994). Foucault (1994) argued that societies surveil and punish certain bodies for the purpose of maintaining social order and exerting control—the female body in our situation (McLaren, 2002).

In doing a discursive analysis such as ours, we must examine "*bodies* of texts because it is the interrelations between texts, changes in texts, new textual forms, and new systems of distributing texts that constitute a discourse over time" (Phillips & Hardy, 2002, p. 5). We will examine a body of texts, including institutional, medical, scientific, popular press, mediated sources, and personal stories to reveal the ways in which the *power behind* (Fairclough, 1989) the pro-breastfeeding discourse has constrained women's choices and created a social reality that privileges some and silences others while disciplining *all*.

The bodies of texts relate to Foucault's (2010b) concept of orders of discourse. For Fairclough (1996), orders of discourse are "the structured set of discursive practices—of different discourses and different genres—associated with a particular social space" (p. 286). He further suggests that, with any discursive analysis which focuses on discourses attempting to shape or reshape practices, a critic must engage the discourse with a dual orientation of both rhetorical and discursive approaches (Fairclough, 1996). In short, we need to look at the event, its rhetorical challenges, and the order of discourses that are utilized to understand how the knowledge and power embedded in the discourses function.

In sum, hegemonic mothering is the result of a variety of discourses that have been structured and ordered in such a way that they cohere around one shared ideology: breast milk is the only acceptable form of infant nutrition. In chapter 2, we start our analysis by describing the socio-cultural discourses of each of the different eras (1950s to today) that set the backdrop for understanding the subsequent actions related to the breast-is-best movement. Chapter 3 contains the results of a close textual read of five key texts and corresponding initiatives that have led to the birth of the medicalization and institutionalization of breastfeeding. The pregnancy and childbirth genre of popular press books are analyzed in chapter 4 and race, class, and white privilege are interrogated in chapter

5. Before examining several mediated examples and blogging mom's voice of resistance as well as drawing our book to its conclusion in chapter 7, we "hear" in chapter 6 the voices of parents that we know who have lived this experience. These discourses represent interdependent networks, structures, or orders of discourse (Fairclaugh, 1989; Foucault, 1984) which have worked together to form what we have labeled the breast-is-best discursive formation. Figure 1.1 captures the interdependent discourses and key processes that form the breast-is-best discursive formation and, in turn, hegemonic motherhood.

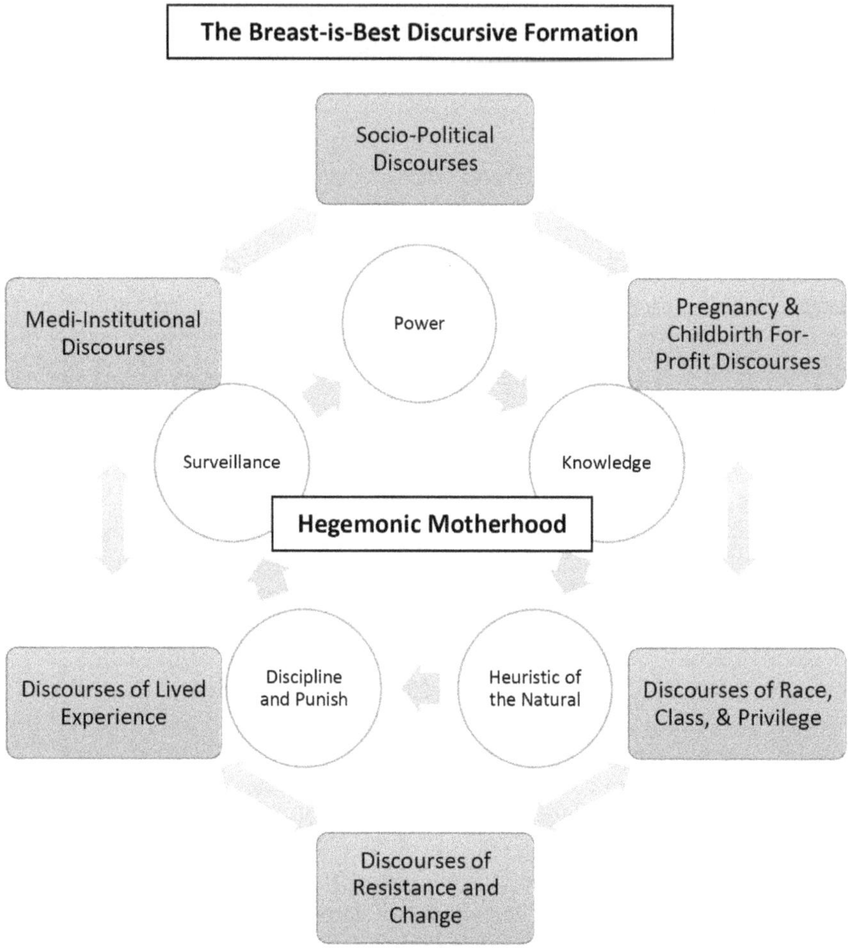

Figure 1.1. The Breast-is-Best Discursive Formation. Created by author.

We realize that this archaeological approach to the breastfeeding discourse will most likely upset many who ascribe to the breast-is-best ideology. It is not a popular endeavor to criticize the breast-is-best coda, or, in other words, to not abide by the scriptures of the gospel of the breast. Yet the archaeologist's task is to break down boundaries and to question taken-for-granted assumptions. Our job is "not in making clarity but in making strange. It consists not in providing definitive answers but in raising more questions" (Radford, 2003, pp. 16–17). We certainly hope that many questions and conversations will occur as you read the coming pages. Importantly, like the parents who bravely share their personal stories about formula feeding their babies (see chapter 6), we believe that some who read our words may find comfort in knowing they are not alone. Many other mothers and parents have walked this same path. One that today is often filled with harsh judgment. It is our hope that the examination of the ideology of the pro-breastfeeding movement through a feminist lens allows us to examine the (dis)empowering way in which breastfeeding is framed. By exposing the ideological constraints embedded in a variety of discourses that thwart their attempts to define motherhood for themselves, this book can play a role in mothers' abilities to take back their freedom of choice. *Our goal is not to dissuade women from breastfeeding their babies, but instead to help create a "space" where all choices are valued, recognizing that all "feeding choices are socially situated"* (Wolf, 2013, p. 309).

TWO

Building the Breast-is-Best Discursive Formation

A Genealogy of Hegemonic Motherhood

The history of breastfeeding in America is a story of influence over women, their bodies, their babies, and a mother's autonomy. Unpacking that history reveals discourses of power, reminiscent of Foucault (1972; 1979) as well as feminist appropriations of Foucault (e.g., McLauren, 2002), that stem from cultural narratives of gender, economics, politics, religion, medicine, and science. At different socio-historical periods, these narratives have intermingled in specific ways to adjudicate women's breastfeeding practices in the United States (Thulier, 2009). Feeding practices have sometimes been articulated in terms of what is best for the baby—sometimes even what is best for the father. What breastfeeding narratives have rarely—if ever—been about is what is best for the mother. This chapter examines the discourses that influence the "reality" of breastfeeding in the United States. Whether breastfeeding, bottle feeding, wet-nursing, or otherwise, women's choice, their right, and their ability to nourish their baby in ways that are best for their infants, their family, and themselves, has never been the "heart" of the conversation. Even when well intentioned, breastfeeding narratives have served as discourses of power and control. In this chapter, we look at the concept of discursive formations as explained by Foucault (1972; 1979) to reveal the essentialist narratives that oversee the "truth" of infant feeding in the United States (and arguably, around the world). For Foucault (2010a), "whenever, between objects, types of statement, concepts, or thematic choices, one can define a regularity (an order . . .), we will say, for the sake of convenience, that we are dealing with a *discursive formation*" (p. 38).

Discursive formations, generally speaking, are the systems of knowledge that are created via texts, statements, objects, etc., that govern ways of thinking (and thus behavior) in a given historical time period (Foucault, 1979). For Foucault, language creates truth. Hall (2001) explains:

> It [language] defines and produces the objects of our knowledge. It governs the way that a topic can be meaningfully talked about and reasoned about. It also influences how ideas are put into practice and used to regulate the conduct of others. Just as a discourse "rules in" certain ways of talking about a topic, defining an acceptable and intelligible way to talk, write, or conduct oneself, so also, by definition, it "rules out," limits and restricts other ways of talking, of conducting ourselves in relation to the topic or constructing knowledge about it. (p. 72)

Foucault was particularly interested in how various discourses create systems of meaning, and in turn, shape the "truth" of how we act in and organize our social world (Foucault, 1972). According to Dreyfus and Rabinow (1982), discursive formations police the minds and bodies of individual actors (everyday people). Accordingly, we look at the discursive formations that police infant feeding via discipline, absence, and, importantly for Foucault, punishment. For as Judith Butler (2004) argues, "it is through the body that gender and sexuality become exposed to others, implicated in social processes, inscribed by cultural norms, and apprehended in their social meanings" (p. 20).

All discourses are part of a "discursive field" of language, social institutions, and systems of power (Foucault, 1972). Our criticism follows McGee's (1980) method of linking these discursive fields, or in McGee's terms, disparate texts, to reveal the hegemonic web that shapes reality. In this case, laws/government, education, religion, medical discourse, socioeconomic changes, and popular culture weave the web of knowledge around breastfeeding. The following discussion details trends in breastfeeding, laws, political ideology, governmental actions, and labor statistics to define the parameters of breastfeeding's discursive field. The formations we've isolated here coalesce, intermingle, and construct what we are calling hegemonic motherhood. Underlying each formation are traditional gender norms that bind women to reproduction and parenting. Women's social realities are thus tied to their children, and, as Blume (1999) articulates, the result is an intense and exclusively feminine internal struggle where women fear being replaced. Our social value diminishes without our exclusive ties to our children. Our power is placed in our biological abilities to feed and care for those children, should we choose to bare them.

Our analysis is particularly interested in the discursive formations that have shaped our realities as mothers since the latter half of the twentieth century. To harken Foucault's (1972) genealogy of discourse, the sections follow a chronological timeline that supports and leads to what we have labeled *the Breast-is-Best Discursive Formation*, beginning with the very late 1940s and into the 1950s. Each formation is situated within its socio-historical *and* political context to develop a framework of social attitudes, beliefs, and discourses. Among the discourses over the last seventy years are common threads of conservatism in politics, religion, and gender, and a "heuristic of the natural," or the belief that a return to the "inherent" biological "purpose" of humans—in particular, women—produces healthier children.

BUILDING THE BREAST-IS-BEST DISCURSIVE FORMATION

Field of Discourses: The Pill, the Baby Bottle, and the Rise in Conservatism (1940s–1960s)

Timeline of Important Events

1. 1946—Bottles become easier to produce and manufacture using plastics technology developed during World War II.[1]
2. The AMA recognizes birth control as a new sector of medical practice and education.[2]
3. 1948—Planned Parenthood helps fund the development and testing of "the pill" by research biologist, Gregory Pincus.[3]
4. 1946–1950—Breastfeeding rates drop to only 25 percent initiation.[4]
5. 1956—The Business and Professional Women Foundation is created to "provide research information, career development programs, and scholarships to disadvantaged women, workshops and other training opportunities."[5]
6. 1956—La Leche League forms. Promotes natural motherhood, cultural feminism, and breastfeeding.[6]
7. 1960—The U.S. Food and Drug Administration approves the sale of oral pills for contraception.[7]
8. 1961—Presidential Committee on the Status of Women is created to explore women's role in the labor force.[8]
9. 1963—Equal Pay Act is passed.[9]
10. *Griswold v. Connecticut*: The Supreme Court nullified a Connecticut statute prohibiting the use of birth control by married persons. The new law argued that married individuals have privacy rights that protect their access to contraceptives.[10]
11. Title VII of the Civil Rights Act of 1964: federal law that prohibits employers from discriminating against employees on the basis of sex, race, color, national origin, and religion.[11]
12. 1965—One in every five married women in the United States has used the pill.[12]

13. 1966—The National Organization for Women is founded by Betty Friedan.[13]

The Era's Discourses of Unity

The social developments of the 1950s and 1960s illustrate the correlation between breastfeeding rates and women's autonomy (Wright & Schanler, 2001). Women in the 1950s and 1960s experienced new developments in reproductive health that coincided with better labor laws and opportunities for employment. The definition of "woman" was no longer limited to "mother." There were other options for women, or perhaps more appropriately—more options—in addition to their roles in the home. While the timeline above is the black and white version of social upheaval, it's the discursive spaces happening within these lines that created other ways of knowing. The unraveling of traditional gender roles revealed just how tightly we organized (and continue to organize) our lives, attitudes, and beliefs around gender.

Women's reproductive and employment rights are part of a discursive framework that allowed society to understand women differently. As a result, since the 1950s, the science of breastfeeding has been connected to labor and the workforce. The advent of modern bottle feeding and formulas provided women with a choice and gave them a sense of agency. Women's participation in the workforce subsequently rose to 34 percent in 1950 and by the late 1950s, most babies were formula fed (Ryan, Pratt, Wysong, Lewandowski, McNally, & Krieger, 1991, p. 1050). In the 1960s, government agencies and institutions began to monitor the formula industry. In 1967, "The American Academy of Pediatrics Committee on Nutrition first made recommendations for vitamins and mineral levels for infant formulas" (Shuman, 2003, p. 92). Women were linked together via the medical community and the government. Each had taken a vested interest—for multiple reasons—in alternative infant feeding practices. Regardless of their intentions, the rise in bottle feeding during this period is a product of interworking discourses. While even early research showed there were some benefits to breastfeeding, they also demonstrated that in wealthy countries, artificial formulas were a safe alternative to breastfeeding. Formula feeding was "ruled in" (in Hall's terms) as an appropriate way "of conducting oneself" (which is a result of a discursive formation).

While these developments were encouraging for women in general, and feminists in particular, most social change is met with some degree of "backlash" or attempts to dismantle the progress gained by subordinate groups (see, for example, McRobbie, 2004). Throughout the latter half of the twentieth century, the dominant discordant discourse seeking to dismantle women's social progress was situated in conservative political ideologies. In the 1950s and 1960s, these discourses were less coordinated than later decades, but nonetheless present in anti-bottle feeding discourses.

The Era's Discourses of Division

During this time period there was a rising tide of American conservatism. American conservatism is marked by a tenuous relationship between moral traditionalists and "free market" classic liberals (Schneider, 2003). Throughout the 1950s (and as we explain later, significantly in the 1980s), these two groups increasingly interacted to shape modern conservatism (Foust, 2008). Conservatism in the United States is itself a discursive formation and its own genealogical project, which has been thoroughly studied by political, historical and communication scholars alike (see, for example, Smith, 2017). For our project, we look at the rise of conservatism that began after World War II in response to shifting geopolitical alliances and the rise of Communism. Smith (2017) explains:

> Prior to Eisenhower's ascendancy, conservatives were energized by various events. In 1948, Undersecretary of State Alger Hiss, who attended the Yalta conference and helped to form the United Nations, was found to have been a member of a communist club. In 1949, China fell to Mao Zedong and the Soviet Union exploded an atomic bomb. In 1950, the United States headed a "police action" in Korea that led to a stalemate. In 1953, alleged spies for the Soviet Union were executed. Throughout this period, Americans were looking for explanations. (p. 37)

Conservatives played off of fear and paranoia to provide those explanations (Smith, 2017). But, rhetoric of fear isn't sustainable, and the Republican party would split between moral traditionalists and moderates. In the 1960s, Senator Barry Goldwater began the work of bringing disparate conservative groups together (PBS Learning Media), a move that helped elect Richard Nixon in 1968. So, while conservatism of the period was fractured, it was a potent detractor to women's liberation (which, we argue, includes our choice in feeding our children). Phyllis Schlafly, for example, an ardent opponent of women's rights, argued for a return to the "True Women" (Solomon, 1979). Schlafly employed conservative discourses to romanticize a woman's journey through married life and motherhood. She acknowledged the frustrations that come with motherhood, but portrayed them as the necessary frustrations inherent to any journey. The difficulties of motherhood were simply part of being a True Woman (Solomon, 1979). Conservative discourses like Schlafly's romanticized motherhood by creating a feminist guise where a woman's role as a caregiver indirectly provided her with power. "The image of women in traditional contexts as dynamic and self-directed and important," became a vital tenet of hegemonic femininity and was bolstered through other conservative discourses (Solomon, 1979). Organizations, like the La

Leche League, formed around these discourses and were effectively able to "operationalize" hegemonic femininity by embracing the archetypal True Woman and exploiting the "natural beauty" of her being.

"Nature," or what is "natural" to the human body fueled conservative discourses against bottle feeding. Nadesan and Sotirin (1998) explain "that maternal breastfeeding by upper-class women most often occurs during historical periods in which dominant social discourses afford a privileged and romanticized status to 'nature'" (p. 219). Cultural attitudes in the latter half of the twentieth century sought a return to "the natural," fueled by a belief that our ailing bodies, are at least in part, a product of what we eat. "The Heuristic of the Natural," as we have termed it, is a revival of natural living practices that Western societies employ as a means to bring the benefits of agrarian living into the modern household.

Heuristics "simplify decision-making through a process of attribute substitution; in other words, they enable users to solve a complex problem by substituting a similar but simpler problem" (McGeough & Rudick, 2018, p. 168). In short, heuristics allow people to problem solve on their own without having to consult experts or expert research. They provide mental short cuts to solutions, particularly for things we fear (Niewert, 2017). For years, medical practitioners controlled knowledge, and as gatekeepers, shaped discourses of the body for much of the twentieth century. Second-wave feminism, however, challenged the patriarchal order of medicine (Largo Janssen, 2007). Feminists decried medical research that only focused on male bodies (Travis, 1993). They also fought to create spaces for women in medical school. Their efforts would *eventually* change the medical profession, but even early on, second-wave feminism challenged dominating medical discourses: "Starting after 1968, this second wave of feminism was responsible for encouraging women to develop their own knowledge and understanding. Women were encouraged to challenge medical power, control things for themselves, and avoid unnecessary medical interventions" (Thulier, 2009, p. 90).

However, second-wave feminism, like all social movements was not a monolithic social construction. The movement's dominant discourses (liberal feminist discourses) competed with other feminist commitments, particularly cultural feminism. Cultural feminists, such as Shafley, found woman's power in her ability to nurture and care, and largely sought to gain more cultural acceptance of womanly attributes. Much like the Cult of True Womanhood, cultural feminists of the latter half of the twentieth century and beginning of the twenty-first century also engaged in heuristics of the natural, but for very different outcomes.

The La Leche League International (LLLI) is an example of a cultural feminist organization that found footing in this era of contentious gendered negotiation, and over the years, has had an enormous effect on how mothers feed their children. LLLI originated in 1956 as part of a Catholic push toward natural and moralistic family living (Ember & Ember, 2003). LLLI was created in Franklin Park, Illinois, by Mary White, Edwina Froehlich, Mary Cahill, Betty Spandikow, Viola Lennon, Mary Kerwin, and Marian Tompson (LLLI: Biographical information, 2011b). Each were married with children and their families were active in the Christian Family Movement, "a national network of parish/neighborhood small groups of families. Parents meet regularly in one another's homes . . . Christian values are reinforced and families are encouraged to reach out in action to others" (Christian Family Movement, 2009). LLLI's founders identified as cultural feminists who believed, that "women should reclaim control of their bodies through natural childbirth and breastfeeding" (Bobel, 2001, p. 135).

In 1958, LLLI published the first edition of *The Womanly Art of Breastfeeding*, a conical text used to promote the importance of breastfeeding. In 1960, the first LLLI group was founded outside the United States in Jonquiere, Quebec, and by 1964 the group was operating globally ("A brief history of," 2011a). By the end of the 1960s, LLLI had found a seat at the international table and was wielding significant influence over breastfeeding narratives. With added awareness of and participation in the organization, breastfeeding rates started to climb. They jumped 4 percent in 1971 and would continue to grow at a rate of 3 percent throughout the rest of the decade. LLLI's persistence and ability to mobilize had changed breastfeeding narratives and would continue to play an important role as the organization mapped itself into medical and scientific discourses.

To summarize the era, the discursive formations of the 1940s, 1950s, and 1960s were marked by technological advances in infant feeding, most notably formula and the rubber nipple. Socially, women were granted more autonomy with the advent of the birth control pill, however, that autonomy was checked by a conservative backlash that sought to maintain a traditional gendered order. In turning to the 1970s and 1980s, discursive formations of motherhood and breastfeeding would follow a similar ebb and flow between medical and social advances, and conservative checks and balances.

Field of Discourses: Our Body, Ourselves', or the Government's? (1970s–1980s)

Timeline of Important Events

1. 1970—Congress passes and President Nixon signs into law Title X of the Public Health Service Act. Title X makes contraceptives available to everyone regardless of income and provides funding for educational programs and research in contraceptive development. Congress broadens Title X's mandate to provide commu-

nity-based sex education programs and preventive services to teenagers at risk of becoming pregnant.[14]

2. 1970—50,000 women in New York and an estimated 100,000 women nationwide march in the Women's Strike for Equality. The march celebrates the 50th anniversary of the Nineteenth Amendment.[15]
3. 1971—Comprehensive Child Development Act is passed by Congress to insure adequate day care facilities for working families. President Nixon vetoes the bill.[16]
4. 1971—Breastfeeding rate on record: only 25 percent of mothers breastfed their infants amid major cultural shifts occurring in the country. The low rate is attributed to working mothers.[17]
5. 1972—Title IX forbids sexual discrimination in educational settings.[18]
6. 1973: "Babies Mean Business" is published. Critiques infant formula companies of exploiting mothers, particularly in the "Third World."[19]
7. 1973—*Roe v. Wade*: The U.S. Supreme Court ruled against a Texas law prohibiting abortions not necessary to save the woman's life. For the first time women are given a fundamental right to choose.[20]
8. 1974: "Baby Killer" is published. Furthers the arguments, particularly against Nestle, concerning formula feeding in underdeveloped countries.
9. 1976—*Planned Parenthood of Central Missouri v. Danforth*: Court case in which a Missouri statute that required married women have written consent from their husband before obtaining an abortion was overturned. Additionally, minors were no longer required to have written consent from their parents.[21]
10. 1978—Pregnancy Discrimination Act is passed. Amends Title VII of the 1964 Civil Rights Act to include pregnancy in anti-discrimination law.[22]
11. 1980—Breastfeeding initiation begins to increase from 33.4 percent to 54 percent in 1980, and subsequently to 59.7 percent in 1984.[23]
12. 1981—The International Code of Marketing of Breast-milk Substitutes is adopted.
13. 1981—Adolescent Family Life Act is passed, funding chastity only sexual educational programs.[24]
14. 1982—Breastfeeding rate jumps to 62 percent.[25]
15. The Guttmacher Institute reveals that the US teen pregnancy rate of 96 per 1,000 is the highest among developed nations.[26]
16. 1985—1986—Anti-family planning groups begin their campaign of "Year of Pain and Fear."[27]
17. 1983—1989—Family Planning clinics are fire bombed and vandalized, clinic staff are assaulted and abortion doctors are sent death

threats. Planned Parenthood clinics on the east coast are targets of arson, bombs, and other violence.[28]

18. 1988—The International Society for Research in Human Milk and Lactation is formed.[29]
19. 1988—Reagan implements Title X gage rule which bars medical professionals from providing information on abortion as a method of family planning.[30]
20. 1989—The Planned Parenthood Action Fund is formed and quickly engages in public education campaigns, grassroots organizing, and legislative advocacy.[31]
21. 1989—U.S. Surgeon General's Workshop rearticulates the benefits of breastfeeding and lactation experts.[32]

Discourses of Contention

The 1970s and 1980s might be best described as a complicated "tug of war" between social attitudes toward women and reproduction. Backlash to women's rights movements found footing in the political rhetoric of the 1970s which intensified in 1980s. Conservative attitudes took hold as society began to feel the "hangover" of the 1960s. While feminist movements continued to gather strength, the 1970s was marked by a frustrating two step of gains and losses. Hauser (2012) explains the cultural atmosphere of the era:

> "You've come a long way, baby," was another popular saying of that era, which originated on cigarette advertisements meant to acknowledge the giant strides of the women's movement . . . But judging from a January 1975 article in *Personnel Journal*, the forebear of *Workforce Management*, some of the concepts embraced by the women's movement, including equality in the workplace and the C-suite, were not going over well in tradition-bound workplaces. (para. 6–7)

Women lived in a contested reality of progress and traditionalism. Through an amalgam of conservative discourses, heuristics of the natural, medical discourse and governmental oversight, breastfeeding regained some popularity. Like breastfeeding discourses today, many of those advocating for breastfeeding were both pro-mothers and pro-babies. But some, as we argue in this section, were far more interested in exclusive breastfeeding as a means to keep women in the home.

Discourses of Surveillance and Traditionalism

All governmental policies are created through a complex system of social attitudes and beliefs. Their result or enactment is rarely, if ever, without some unintended (although certainly intended by some) consequences. In terms of gender, Baer (2016) explains that there is a "double nature of norms governing gender, which both constrain and enable life"

(p. 23). An example of this is the 1979 U.S. Surgeon General's report entitled "Healthy People Objectives for 1990." This action set a series of national targets for infant health and breastfeeding:

> Human breast milk provides nutritionally complete, convenient, pre-warmed food for infants. Breastfeeding also increases mother-infant contact, confers some protection from infectious diseases by transferring antibodies from mother to child, and helps women who have gained excessive weight during pregnancy to lose it. Moreover, breast fed infants rarely are obese and virtually never develop iron deficiency anemia, the most common nutritional problem of American infants. If the nursing mother is healthy and well fed, fluoride and possibly vitamin D may be the only supplements needed by the baby. After about four months, a source of iron may also have to be added to the diet. Commercial formulas are available and when prepared according to direction provide adequate nutrition but, in contrast to breastfeeding, they are not regarded as the optimal food source. (U.S. Department of Health and Human Services, 1979, pp. 14–15)

In 1984, the Surgeon General's office intensified its efforts to encourage breastfeeding via the U.S. Department of Health and Human Services. The latter instituted serial publications, some of which are the focus of chapter 3, and workshops specifically designed to increase breastfeeding rates in the United States (Brown, Bair, & Meier, 2003).

As read, the laws and objectives passed in the 1970s support the health and well-being of infants and demonstrate some of the government's first public awareness of women and our needs as mothers and individuals. But, government involvement in breastfeeding coincided and was influenced by a number of social contributors. LLLI was one of these groups. Their increasing presence in national discussions of women's health played an increasingly powerful role in shaping breastfeeding discourses.

As previously mentioned, LLLI was one of the religious groups that supported women, but primarily from a traditionalist standpoint that was at odds with women's liberation. In the 1970s and 1980s, the organization's star began to rise. In 1971 Princess Grace of Monaco spoke at the organization's 4th International Conference. That same year, with more awareness of, and participation in the organization, breastfeeding rates rose 4 percent. They continued an average climb of 3 percent throughout the rest of the decade. In 1979 the organization was part the joint WHO/UNICEF meeting on Infant and Young Child Feeding in Geneva, Switzerland ("A brief history of," 2011a), and UNCIF, in 1981, gave LLLI consultative status. An updated version of *The Womanly Art of Breastfeeding* was also published in 1981 to coincide with the 25th anniversary of the International Conference ("A brief history of," 2011a). Breastfeeding initiation rates continued to rise, and in 1982 they reached 61.9 percent. In 1987, the Peer Counselor Program where mothers mentor and counsel other mothers on breastfeeding was created. The Center for Breastfeeding information (CBI), which is considered the world's largest resource for scientific research on breastfeeding, was established along with an 800-line to allow mothers to reach out to other LLLI groups ("A brief history of," 2011a). LLLI's rise throughout the 1970s and 1980s is an impressive example of organizing and marketing, but its ability to thrive is arguably attributed to the conservative political tides that rose in the 1950s and 1960s that once again flourished in the 1980s.

The Continued Rise of Conservatism in the 1980s

Tenets of the religious right (a conservative subgroup we examine more closely in the discursive political formations of the 1980s) can be traced, arguably to America's puritan beginnings, but the landmark Supreme Court decision on *Roe v. Wade* united the already formidable protestant movement with other religious groups (most notably Catholics and Orthodox Jews) (McVicar, 2016). They would build a discursive religious framework supported by politics and implemented by laws. In the 1970s and 1980s, they relied on the natural, biological—and thus Christian—roles of women (which included breastfeeding) to fight abortion and other reproductive rights. In politics and law, men have historically led policy making, even in regard to women's bodies. While many women support conservative ideologies, underrepresentation of women in congress created a void—a presence of absence—for alternative views on women's rights. So while there were a number of gains for women in the 1970s and 1980s, there were also subversive groups—particularly religious groups—working against women's autonomy under a feminist guise that touted power through natural mothering.

While conservative political attitudes had been on the rise, in some form or another, since World War II, it was Ronald Regan who bridged the rhetorical divide between competing conservative ideologies using stories of "everyday heroes" that came from all walks of life (Shogun, 2006, p. 220). His ability to unify the Republican party shaped conservatism until the populist movement in 2016. Reagan's rhetoric is important here, because it is an example of discursive formations molding common sense realities of the everyday citizen:

> With his stories and parables, Reagan deliberately targeted listeners as individuals rather than as a collective entity. Reagan spoke directly to each citizen, with the goal that his speeches could change their actions and decisions. (Shogun, 2006, p. 220)

Reagan colored his economic rhetoric with religious undertones in order to unite his audience (free marketers and moral traditionalists) in a common cause. Shogun (2006) explains that Reagan's rhetoric took on a conservative "theme" where voters were told "the nation's economic situation teetered on the edge of disaster unless citizens repented and reformed. The recovery of the economy depended upon the American people exhibiting a 'quasi-religious faith' in the president's policies and programs" (p. 223). Reagan's reliance on faith, and a willingness—if not eagerness—to bring faith back into the White House, helped establish a discursive field where politics and religion would once again dictate the lives of everyday people. At the National Affairs briefing conference—a rally for a huge coalition of Christians, young and old—Reagan cemented the relationship between U.S. policy and Christian teachings by famously stating, "I know you can't endorse me, but I endorse you and what you are doing" (McVicar, 2016).

Throughout Reagan's two terms in office, moral evangelists provided the president insight and guidance that shaped U.S. laws and practices (Zoll, 2007). Reagan sought to reinstate moral virtues of the family, which included the unborn. Abortion law, in particular, drove political and religious zealotry that sought to limit reproductive rights, and implicitly, if not explicitly (see Jimmy Swaggart, for example) return women to the home. The line between Church and State blurred as politicians and religious leaders fought to diminish the effects of *Roe v. Wade.* If they couldn't overturn it, they would fervently work to limit it. Zoll (2007) nicely sums up the relationship between religious leaders and politicians of the time: "It may be hard to remember now, but conservative preachers avoided politics in the days when Falwell began his ministry. Then the U.S. Supreme Court legalized abortion in 1973" (Washingtonpost.com). The mission of many became saving babies at all costs, including the cost of their mothers.

This was perhaps most evident with the Religious (or Christian) right, which "refers to a loose network of political actors, religious organizations, and political pressure groups that formed in the United States in the late 1970s" (McVicar, 2016, p. 1). While President Carter utilized these groups in relation to his strong, Southern Baptist faith, it was President Reagan who invited them into the White House. The Religious Right adopted a "grassroots" (we use this term with some skepticism, since the religious right would become a corporate entity with millions of dollars and vast political influence) strategy of recruiting voters and would eventually drive policy discussions well into the 2000s (McVicar, 2016). They would be the motivating force behind religious and political life for conservatives in the United States (McVicar, 2016).

Jerry Falwell and Pat Robertson were two of the most prominent faces of the Religious Right Movement. Falwell was a Baptist preacher, televangelist, the creator of Liberty University, and the founder of the Moral Majority. "As much as anyone, he helped create the religious right as a political force, defined the issues that would energize it for decades and cemented its ties to the Republican party" (Applebome, 2007, para. 6). The Moral Majority set out to build "a coalition of these different religious groups that all agree on abortion and homosexuality and other issues even if they never agreed on how to read the Bible or the nature of God" (John Green as cited in Applebome, 2007, para. 9). In the 1970s, Falwell confronted an American culture that, as he saw it, was in moral free fall. His work sparked a mass movement that transformed the Republican Party, conservative discourse, and U.S. politics.

President Reagan courted Falwell and his allies, recognizing their political influences on large swaths of American voters (Zoll, 2007). Falwell's famous quote: "Get them saved, baptized and registered" (National Broadcasting Company, Nightly News, 1984) was influential in Reagan's 1980 election (Applebome, 2007). Falwell couldn't reverse *Roe v. Wade,* but he did become a fixture in the Reagan White House. He would go on to advise President George W. Bush, and according to Zoll (2007), "GOP political candidates sought his backing and, in later years, treated him as an elder statesman of the party" (Washingtonpost.com).

M. G. "Pat" Robertson, a contemporary of Falwell's, rose in prominence during the same time period. His life has been spent as a:

> religious broadcaster, philanthropist, educator, religious leader, businessman and author. He is the founder and chairman of The Christian Broadcasting Network (CBN) Inc. and founder of International Family Entertainment Inc., Regent University, Operation Blessing International Relief and Development Corporation, American Center for Law and Justice, The Flying Hospital, Inc., and several other organizations and broadcast entities. (The Official Site of Pat Robertson, Biography, para 1)

Robertson ran for president in 1988, but failed to win the Republican party nomination. Nonetheless, Robertson, like Falwell, played an important role in shaping political agendas, particularly in regard to traditional family values and abortion.

The 1970s and 1980s were an era where unlikely and unwitting allies worked in conjunction to roll back women's autonomy in the public sphere. President Reagan brought Protestants, Jews, and Catholics together with help from the Religious Right. Religion once again shaped the political landscape and laws and regulations began to take on conservative tones. While often at odds with each other, these entities and organizations like LLLI, who genuinely seek to help women, found success working within a conservative discursive framework established as an answer to women's liberation. Moreover, the rampant, visceral desire of some religious leaders and politicians to overturn *Roe v. Wade* created fertile ground for conservative ideologies to thrive. Laws that ensured women's fair treatment in the workplace couldn't change the opinion of many that they didn't belong there. For many, women had abandoned their babies and their men for the materialistic world. Conservative discourses sought to shame women back into the home. They added pressure to new mothers to breastfeed and elevated the heuristic of the natural. Then, a horrific international scandal marred the formula industry and seemingly gave credence to conservative beliefs of natural motherhood.

A Discourse of Disruption: The Nestle Scandal

On July 7th, 1977, the United States launched a boycott of Nestle Corporation in response to their aggressive advertising campaigns in Third World countries, particularly those in Africa, that resulted in the malnutrition and deaths of thousands of children. Nestle was accused of: 1) "creating a need where none existed"; 2) "Convincing consumers the products were indispensable"; and 3) "Linking products with the most desirable and unattainable concepts—then giving a sample" (Krasny 2012). To lend credence to their advertising, Nestle hired women—who were not members of the medical community—to sell formula while dressed in nursing uniforms.

The problem was not the formula itself. It was the fact that the water needed to mix the formula was unsafe, resulting in infant death and illness. Additionally, formula was expensive. Mothers who believed the formula could save their babies would reduce the amount of formula they used in each serving in an effort to extend the formula for as long as possible. Babies became sick and died of malnourishment. These women had been led to believe their natural milk was insufficient. They were scared to breastfeed, and they couldn't afford the formula that was supposed to save their children from the fate of living in a poor nation.

The books *Babies Mean Business* and *Baby Killer* brought the scandal to the developed world. Action was swift. In 1975, Nestle filed a libel suit to address the claims made against them. They ultimately won the case, but the fine against the offending company was minimal. In 1978, Senator Kennedy held congressional hearings on the marketing of infant formulas in underdeveloped countries, and in 1979, WHO/UNICEF passed the International Code of Marketing of Breast-milk Substitutes to protect underdeveloped countries from the predatory practices of the formula industry.

While Nestle engaged in egregious acts against mothers and children, the problem with formulas didn't extend to developed countries. Women in the United States could safely feed their children with formula, but the stigma attached to the scandal bolstered anti-bottle feeding discourses. Companies had lied and swindled innocent mothers. They couldn't be trusted to treat women in developed countries any better.

In all, the 1980s were a difficult time for women. While work rates increased, attitudes towards women in the workforce were far from overwhelmingly positive. Women faced a no-win double-bind between staying at home and going to work, and their bodies had become a legal battle ground for reproduction. As a result, discourses of motherhood pulled women in opposite directions. They existed in a limbo of the double-bind, pulled between liberal discourses of autonomy and the conservative discourses fervently working to return women to the home. However, if the 1980s were a response to the social changes of the 1960s and 1970s, the 1990s would bring *some* relief.

Fields of Discourse: The Year of the Woman vs. the Moral Majority (1990s—2000s)

Timeline of Important Events

- 1991—Innocenti Declaration on the Protection, Promotion, and Support of Breastfeeding is created.
- 1992—*Planned Parenthood of Southeastern Pennsylvania v. Casey*: The Supreme Court does not overturn *Roe v. Wade,* however they add strict restrictions for obtaining abortions including parental consent, pre-abortion counseling, and a wait period.[33]
- "The Year of the Woman." Fifty-six women are elected to Congress, more than ever before, thanks in large part to efforts by women's pro-choice PACs.[34]
- 1993—President Bill Clinton, the first pro-choice president in 12 years, is voted into office. In one of his first acts, he repeals the Reagan era Title X gag rule, which prohibited low-income patients from receiving medical information, counseling, or referrals for abortion services. Clinton also overturns the global gag rule that denied funding to international family planning organizations.[35]
- 1993 enactment of the Family and Medical Leave Act.
- President Clinton vetoes two federal abortion bans, one of which stated under federal legislation that physicians could have been jailed, fined, and/or sued for performing safe abortion procedures.[36]
- The "Year of Terror" campaign returns and two abortion provider MD's are killed by anti-abortion zealots.[37]
- 1995—Data reveals that "between 1971 and 1995, increases in breastfeeding initiation occurred in all groups for which data are available. In contrast, the increase that occurred between 1984 to 1995 involved those groups that have been less likely to practice breastfeeding, that is, low income women, WIC participants and those with the least education. Breastfeeding also increased between 1984 and 1995 among both African Americans (from 33.3 to 37 percent), and Hispanics (from 53.8 to 61.0 percent), with little change in breastfeeding initiation among Caucasians (from 65.0 to 64.3 percent)."[38]

- 1995—65 percent of practicing pediatricians advocate exclusive breastfeeding for the first month.[39]
- 1994—Formula companies donate breastfeeding literature and free formula samples to pediatric and obstetric offices.[40]
- 2000—The American Academy of Pediatrics formed a Provisional Section on Breastfeeding.[41]
- Healthy People 2000 made numerous recommendations for enabling employed women to breastfeed.[42]

Discourses of Liberation

The 1990s reinstated a number of women friendly social policies. This is at least, in part, due to women's increased presence in politics and government. Prior to the 1990s, there were very few women in Congress. Jeanette Rankin was the first woman elected to Congress in 1917. Rebecca Latimer was elected to the Senate in 1922. Throughout U.S. history, a total of 329 women have served in congress (212 Democrats, 117 Republicans) (Congressional Research Service Reports). Since Rankin and Latimier, women's representation in congress has "increased incrementally, and on a few occasions, decreased" (Congressional Research Service Reports). Anticipation of a feminine breakthrough in congress had been high since the 1970s, but it wasn't until the 1990s that women made substantial gains in the House and Senate.

> The largest increase occurred in the 103rd Congress (1993–1994), when the total number of women in the House and Senate serving at one time rose from 32 in the 102nd Congress to 54, an increase of nearly 69 percent. The 1992 election came to be known popularly as the "Year of the Woman" due to the large electoral increase of women in Congress. (Congressional Research Service Reports)

Just as the Religious Right rose out of a fear of moral corruption, the number of women in congress rose in response to the Moral Majority's attacks on women's rights (History, Art, and Archives: House of Representatives). In 1992, and again in 1994, many women ran on "women's issues," particularly as they related to education and health care. In 1994, women sought to bring both back into the national conversation after funding for the first Gulf War decreased funding for domestic and social issues (History, Art, and Archives: House of Representatives). While women remained (and remain) underrepresented in Congress, the 1990s saw a rise in women's participation in the politics.

Competing Discourses of Motherhood: LLLI in 1990s—Early 2000s

Competing commitments plague all social movements, and feminism is no different. While women ran for congress and made progress in the workplace, other women-centered organizations—some of whom identify as feminist, others that decidedly do not—worked to refocus "women's issues" on motherhood. LLLI was one of these. As such, the 1990s is an interesting decade for examining how competing discursive commitments intertwine while also diverging, creating some social gains while threatening others.

Although LLLI accomplished much during the 1980s, breastfeeding rates dropped to 50 percent in 1990. LLLI pushed on. They expanded their influence within the United Nations and assisted WHO/UNICEF policymakers to create the "Innocenti Declaration on the Protection, Promotion and Support of Breastfeeding," which was signed by 10 United Nations agencies and 32 countries, including the United States ("A brief history of," 2011a). 1991 proved to be another important year for LLLI as they joined other organizations to form the World Alliance for Breastfeeding Action (WABA), "a global network to protect, support, and promote breastfeeding," ("A brief history of," 2011a) and also supported the launching of The Baby-Friendly Hospital Initiative (BFHI) by WHO/UNICEF (Baby-Friendly USA, 2010). We examine several of these initiatives in more depth in chapter 3. In 1992, WABA sponsored the first World Breastfeeding Week with the theme of Baby-Friendly Hospitals, and LLLI sponsored its first World Walk for Breastfeeding ("A brief history of," 2011a). LLLI established a presence on the internet by creating its own website and participated in "Parent Soup on America Online." Breastfeeding initiation rates once again reached almost 60 percent ("A brief history of," 2011a). In 1997, LLLI held their 25th annual Physicians Seminar, the 40th Anniversary of the International Conference and celebrated the 10th Anniversary of the Peer Counselor Program.

At the dawn of the new millennium, LLLI continued to expand. In 2001, Wellstart International donated their library to LLLI, which increased their number of professional journal articles, research studies, and books available from their CBI from 19,000 to 38,000 ("A brief history of," 2011a). Closing out the decade, the tenth edition of *The Womanly Art of Breastfeeding* was published in 2010.

As LLLI increased its research and funding base, breastfeeding discourses concomitantly became more institutionalized. As a result, the act of breastfeeding (and subsequently bottle feeding) was subjected to increased governmental surveillance. This era marked the beginning of quasi-governmental agencies that began to separate women from infant feeding, positioning the latter firmly in the hands of the state. As we suggested in the introduction, breastfeeding discourses have always revealed social power and control over women. This era, and as we argue more fully in the next chapter, marks the shift of power toward governmental policies.

Fields of Discourse: Good Mothers Breastfeed; Bad Ones Do Not (2010s–2020s)

Timeline of Important Events

- 2000—Women in the labor force reaches 60 percent.[43]
- 2001—The Bush administration reinstates the global gag rule. 80,000 women die each year from unsafe and illegal abortion across the globe.[44]
- 2007—The newly ultraconservative Supreme Court overturns the lower court rulings and upholds the abortion ban that President Bush signed into law in 2003.[45]
- 2009—President Obama overturns the global gag rule, ending eight years of policies that have blocked access to basic health care for women worldwide.[46]
- Federal court rulings state that the FDA must make Plan B emergency contraception available over the counter to all women 17 and older.[47]
- Health care reform as we know it today is first introduced.[48]
- The *2011 Surgeon General's Call to Action to Support Breastfeeding* is adopted.

The early years of the twenty-first century continued the trend of governmental control over women's breasts. In regard to breastfeeding, this era was marked by increased monitoring of breastfeeding by the U.S. government. In chapter 3, we examine the various initiatives quasi-governmental agencies launched during this time period, including the Healthy People of 2000, 2010, and 2020 initiatives, which specifically addressed breastfeeding rates in the United States.

Unfortunately, the downward trend of stripping away women's rights has only continued to gain traction during the Trump administration. For example, Human Rights Watch—World Report 2018—lists the following as direct threats to women's human rights:

- Congress dismantles rule to protect family planning funds (Title X) and limits access to reproductive health care. The act targets organizations like Planned Parenthood, who provide affordable access to health care for low income women.
- Congressional proposals continue to undermine the ACA particularly in relation to women's health services, our ability to claim insurance coverage for reproductive health, and looks to cut funding for Medicaid.
- Trump's executive order on "promoting free speech and religious liberty," limits women's access to reproductive health services. It provides for "conscience-based objections" to the preventive-care mandate of the ACA.

- The Trump White House cancels an equal pay initiative for 2018 which would insure companies provided employee compensation information to civil rights enforcement agencies. Employers will no longer be required to "comply with fair pay measures" and can continue with forced arbitration for sexual harassment complaints.
- The Department of Education announced its intention to review and change guidelines on campus sexual assault, notably the Obama-era guidance on Title IX of Education Amendments Act of 1972.
- Texas, Arkansas, Kentucky, Iowa, Tennessee all pass restrictions on abortion and other reproductive health measures.
- Some states increased efforts to deny public family planning funds to providers who also offer abortion services.
- (For a complete list of the concerns listed by Human Rights Watch, please visit: https://www.hrw.org/world-report/2018/country-chapters/united-states#49dda6)

LLLI in 2010–2020: A Continued Campaign for 100 percent Breastfeeding Rates

As the government stripped away women's rights and simultaneously became more involved in the lives of new mothers during the last decade, LLLI continued to increase its ties to UNICEF, the World Health Organization, and the United Nations. LLLI's current mission is, "to help mothers worldwide to breastfeed through mother-to-mother support, encouragement, information, and education, and to promote a better understanding of breastfeeding as an important element in the healthy development of the baby and mother" (La Leche League, Philosophy).

Nadesan and Sotirin's (1998) analysis of LLLI explains that "The League articulates a naturalistic, essentialist view of mothering and breastfeeding that celebrates the moral superiority and natural reproductive capacities of women" (p. 221). According to *The Womanly Art of Breastfeeding*, "the newborn has but three demands: warmth in the arms of its mother, food from her breast, and security in the knowledge of her presence-breastfeeding satisfies all three" (LLLI: Biographical information, 2011b). The text also informs mothers: "Breastfeeding doesn't give you brownie points. It's simply the normal way to raise a baby" (La Leche League International, 2011).

LLLI's influence on breastfeeding over the last seventy years can't and shouldn't be denied. But the organization is an example of discursive tensions that create dialectical understandings of motherhood in terms of "good" and "bad" moms. For example, listed below are the "points" (also known as facts) that support LLLI's philosophy:

- Mothering through breastfeeding is the most natural and effective way of understanding and satisfying the needs of the baby.

- Mother and baby need to be together early and often to establish a satisfying relationship and an adequate milk supply.
- In the early years the baby has an intense need to be with his mother which is as basic as his need for food.
- Human milk is the natural food for babies, uniquely meeting their changing needs.
- For the healthy, full-term baby, breast milk is the only food necessary until the baby shows signs of needing solids, about the middle of the first year after birth.
- Ideally the breastfeeding relationship will continue until the baby outgrows the need.
- Alert and active participation by the mother in childbirth is a help in getting breastfeeding off to a good start.
- Breastfeeding is enhanced and the nursing couple sustained by the loving support, help, and companionship of the baby's father. A father's unique relationship with his baby is an important element in the child's development from early infancy.
- Good nutrition means eating a well-balanced and varied diet of foods in as close to their natural state as possible.
- From infancy on, children need loving guidance which reflects acceptance of their capabilities and sensitivity to their feelings. (La Leche League International, https://www.llli.org/about/philosophy/)

LLLI's points emphasize the intense and involved nature of "good" mothering. Breastfeeding becomes a procedural process of good mothering. However, despite LLLI's accomplishments for increasing mother/infant experiences throughout the world, these "points" reveal the organization's ethnocentric undertones that disregard other cultures, especially when it comes to race and class. In the United States, LLLI membership mostly consists of mothers who are white, middle class, and married—women who are already more likely to breastfeed than their intercultural and socio-economic counterparts (Bobel, 2001, p. 146). The good mother that emerges from these points can afford to stay home. She . . . is also a she. The assumption presented in these points is a family composed of a female "mother" and male "father." This is a heterosexist, biological family manifestation of parenting that excludes the experiences of adoptive, foster, surrogate, and LGBTQ+ family formations. In addition to being heterosexist and heteronormative, breastfeeding discourses are uniquely situated within the realities of the workforce. The breastfeeding mother is not only assumed to be white, heterosexual, and married—she is also situated within the home.

THEN AND NOW: THE GENEALOGY OF HEGEMONIC MOTHERHOOD

As we have discussed in this chapter, the mid-late twentieth century and first two decades of the twenty-first century has seen women's rights grow at a tremendous pace. Along with an increase in reproductive rights, women's work outside of the home has grown substantially. For example, the labor force participation rate of women age 25 to 54 has increased from just below 20 percent in 1948 to 50 percent in 1970 and to more than 70 percent in 2016 (Hipple, 2016). Similarly, labor force participation for mothers with children under three years of age has also increased from approximately 35 percent in 1975 to slightly more than 60 percent in 2015 (Hipple, 2016).

Yet, as women's participation in the workforce has increased so have the attempts to keep her "in her place," or in other words, at home with a baby attached to her breast (if she's a white, heterosexual, middle-class woman). This unsettling trend, along with others discussed in this chapter, coincides with conservative political agendas that are committed to keeping women in the home. Women's rights movements of the 1960s and 1970s brought women back into the workplace after their return to the home following World War II. At the same time, science, medicine, and women's liberation coalesced in making the birth control pill readily available to women around the world. The result of these simultaneous "shocks" to our cultural system was a discourse of motherhood that changed and yet, frustratingly, stayed the same. At the heart of the discourses are definitions of "good" and "bad." It is no coincidence that as science and culture gave women freedom and choice, discourses of power and discipline reemerged to take that choice away.

Motherhood is often represented as the "ultimate expression of womanhood while breastfeeding is represented as the ultimate experience of motherhood" (Nadesan & Sotirin, 1998, p. 221). We see hegemonic motherhood as a counter discursive formation that sought to afford women power, but one that in our view, has negative consequences for women, as it limits our power to our "womanly attributes" and our "natural" capabilities. It also subsumes the mother's needs to her child's. A quick perusal of the words in LLLI's list of "philosophical points" reveals an emphasis of the "natural," "basic," and "unique" role motherhood plays in a woman and child's life. LLLI places these terms in relation to a mother's love for her child. From a rhetorical perspective, LLLI situates a mother's love in direct relation to the natural act of breastfeeding. The dialectical tension, of course, is that mothers who do not breastfeed, or cannot, are unnatural, or perhaps, do not love their children enough. The personal stories we include in chapter 6 support this claim. Whether through intention or simply the reality of dialectical discourse, the heuristic of the natural is exclusive rhetoric. Giving women the power to determine for themselves what is best for their baby is at the "heart" of the heuristic cause. It is not, however, the outcome.

Nadesan and Sotirin (1998) discuss breastfeeding in terms of discursive tensions. "Discursive tensions," they explain, "frame the nature of choice" (Nadesan & Sotirin, 1998, p. 218). Choice is never truly heuristic. It is always set by parameters:

> If, in following Butler, we believe that gender is performative and that it has no ontological status apart from its ultimately contingent "*stylized repetitions of acts*" (40), then the significance of these discourses of breastfeeding stems from their inscriptions and disciplining of maternal bodies. (Nadesan & Sotirin, 1998, p. 217)

We agree with Nadesan and Sotirin (1998) that "breastfeeding is a loaded signifier" (p. 218). We further agree with their claim that:

> Women in Western Culture are confronted with a "choice" between two subjectivities: "womanly power—the nurturing, competent, selfless mother, always sacrificing, the soul of goodness; or the fiery, voluptuous vamp with the power of attraction, leading victims down the road of pleasure, sin and danger." (p. 197)

Women's "choice" to breastfeed is framed by discourses of a natural, moral, and maternal duty, on the one hand, and discourses of the "risky mother" on the other. In gender scholarship, the risky woman is a woman who puts her own needs before others (particularly men and children). She shirks the selflessness (even if momentarily) that "good" mothers possess at all times. A truly "good" mother, is a woman whose gender performance is static. She is "all in" for her children at all times. The heuristic of the natural places women in an unfair dichotomy.

The natural mother remains a selfless woman who sacrifices herself, is a subordinate to male pleasure, and is intensely focused on the needs of her infant. The resulting narrative reinforces the "natural mother as a conservative force, reinforcing prevailing pro-natalist, heterosexual, pro-family, and pro-capitalist social and moral orders" (Nadesan & Sotirin, 1998, pp. 220–21).

Hegemonic motherhood via exclusive mothering discourses limit choice by representing motherhood as a woman's most significant life experience. Exclusive mothering narratives are an example of homogenized discourse that works in conjunction with seemingly disparate texts (government, laws, popular culture, media), with the effect of creating an "ideology of breastfeeding." The natural mother is glorified through women-centered discourse while women who deny their children life-saving/making breast milk are debased, or perhaps more accurately presented as amoral, via the presence of absence. LLLI tells women that "No one else can take your place" (Nadesan & Sotirin, 1998, p. 221). Mothers, at least the good ones, must always be there. Mothers who choose not to breastfeed are literally absent from LLLI discourse, which implies their morals are absent as well.

The lure of exclusive mothering discourses for feminists is seemingly obvious: Exclusive mothering discourses disrupt capitalist ideologies by promoting pro-woman discourse and woman-to-woman interaction and empowerment "against institutionalized male and medical authority" (Nadesan & Sotirin, 1998, p. 222). Enter the pragmatic paradox: There is no question that LLLI and other pro-breastfeeding organizations have been a constant contributor to new laws and statutes that make it possible for women to breastfeed at work and in public. However, the dualistic discourse of natural/pro-woman results in the same tension experienced by Cult feminists throughout women's liberation history. The rhetoric of the choice to breastfeed leaves little actual choice. LLLI and other like-minded organizations resolve the social tensions over breastfeeding through the heuristic of the natural, but in doing so, resituate the woman to her "natural" biological role.

NOTES

1. https://www.alimentarium.org/en/magazine/history/history-baby-bottles.
2. Our Bodies, Our Choices Blogspot. Our Bodies, Our Choices Blogspot. http://obocnow.blogspot.com/2012/04/timeline-of-reproductive-rights.html.
3. Our Bodies, Our Choices Blogspot.
4. Charles Hirschman and Marilyn Butler. (1981). Trends and Differentials on Breastfeeding: An Update. *Demography, 18*, 1, 39–54.
5. Women in Labor History Timeline (https://www.afscme.org/for-members/womens-leadership-training/leadership-tools/body/Women_in_Labor_History_Timeline.pdf).
6. La Leche League International.
7. Our Bodies, Our Choices Blogspot.
8. Executive Order 10980 (December 14, 1961).
9. United States. Department of Labor. Office of the Solicitor. (1963). Legislative history of the Equal Pay Act of 1963, amending section 6 of the Fair Labor Standards Act of 1938, as amended, Public Law 88-38, 88th Congress, H.R. 6060 and S. 1409. Washington: U.S. G.P.O.
10. Our Bodies, Our Choices Blogspot.
11. American Association of University Women. (N/D). "Know Your Rights: Title VII of the Civil Rights Act of 1964." Retrieved from https://www.aauw.org/what-we-do/legal-resources/know-your-rights-at-work/title-vii/.
12. Our Bodies, Our Choices Blogspot.
13. Molly Wolfe. (June 30, 2015). "This day in history: National Organization for Women was founded. The White House Blog. Retreived from https://obamawhitehouse.archives.gov/blog/2015/06/30/day-history-national-organization-women-was-founded.
14. Our Bodies, Our Choices Blogspot.
15. Susan Hauser. (May 15, 2012). "The Women's Movement in the '70s, Today: 'You've Come a Long Way,' But . . . " *Workforce*. Retrieved from https://www.workforce.com/2012/05/15/thewomens-movement-in-the-70s-today-youve-come-a-long-way-but/.
16. Sascha Cohen. (August 26, 2015). "The day women went on strike." *Time Magazine*. Retrieved from http://time.com/4008060/women-strike-equality-1970/.

17. Wright and Schanler. (2001). "The resurgence of breastfeeding."
18. Cohen, (2015). "The day women went on strike."
19. Wright and Schanler. (2001). "The resurgence of breastfeeding."
20. Our Bodies, Our Choices Blogspot.
21. Our Bodies, Our Choices Blogspot.
22. The Pregnancy Discrimination Act, 42 US Code Chapter 21 Sec. 701 (k) of Civil Rights Act of 1964 Title VII. Retrieved from https://www.eeoc.gov/laws/statutes/pregnancy.cfm.
23. Wright and Schanler, (2001), "The resurgence of breastfeeding."
24. Our Bodies, Our Choices Blogspot.
25. Wright and Schanler. (2001). "The resurgence of breastfeeding."
26. Our Bodies, Our Choices Blogspot.
27. Our Bodies, Our Choices Blogspot.
28. Our Bodies, Our Choices Blogspot.
29. Wright and Schanler. (2001). "The resurgence of breastfeeding."
30. National Family Planning and Reproductive Health Association. "Domestic gag rule: Challenges for Title X patients and providers." Retrieved from https://www.nationalfamilyplanning.org/file/Domestic-Gag-Fact-Sheet.pdf.
31. Our Bodies, Our Choices Blogspot.
32. Wright and Schanler. (2001). "The resurgence of breastfeeding."
33. Our Bodies, Our Choices Blogspot.
34. Our Bodies, Our Choices Blogspot.
35. Our Bodies, Our Choices Blogspot.
36. Our Bodies, Our Choices Blogspot.
37. Our Bodies, Our Choices Blogspot.
38. Wright and Schanler. (2001). "The resurgence of breastfeeding."
39. Wright and Schanler. (2001). "The resurgence of breastfeeding."
40. Wright and Schanler. (2001). "The resurgence of breastfeeding."
41. Wright and Schanler. (2001). "The resurgence of breastfeeding."
42. Wright and Schanler. (2001). "The resurgence of breastfeeding."
43. Sandra Black, Diane Whitmore Schanzenbach, and Audrey Breitwieser, A. (2017). "The recent decline in women's labor force participation. *The Hamilton Project.* Retrieved from http://www.hamiltonproject.org/papers/the_recent_decline_in_womens_labor_force_participation.
44. Our Bodies, Our Choices Blogspot.
45. Our Bodies, Our Choices Blogspot.
46. Our Bodies, Our Choices Blogspot.
47. Our Bodies, Our Choices Blogspot.
48. Our Bodies, Our Choices Blogspot.

THREE

Creating the Gaze

The Birth of the Medi-Institionalization of Breastfeeding

Moving in concurrent fashion with the dialectical nature of feminism action and conservatist backlash during the mid-twentieth and early twenty-first centuries, a major goal of governments, global health organizations, hospitals, and governmental public health agencies has been to increase the rate of breastfeeding. As such, we have witnessed the signature of numerous declarations, worldwide initiatives, and U.S. governmental public health "calls to action." There is no doubt that each of these acts, along with those carried out by organizations such as La Leche League, has helped promote breastfeeding, which is certainly a good thing. Yet, as we will argue, such actions have formed the framework for institutionalizing and medicalizing the act of breastfeeding. Similar to Foucault's treatises on the births of the clinic (1994) and prison (1995), we assert that the initiatives, policies, and corresponding documents have led to the *birth of the medicalization and institutionalization of breastfeeding*. This medi-institutional gaze is a convergence of political ideology, institutional legitimacy, and medical authority which has objectified the mother and turned her into a subject who must be observed and disciplined (Foucault, 1994; 1995). As Butler (2004) states of the female body, "the body has its invariably public dimension; constituted as a social phenomenon in the public sphere, my body is, and is not, mine" (p. 21). The medicalization and institutionalization of breastfeeding has constrained mothers' autonomy and, more directly, their bodies, telling them how they were to mother and disciplined them for not doing it the right way—the breastfeeding way.

The documents created and discussed in this chapter enclosed information about breastfeeding in a defined space, creating a form of totalization (Foucault, 1994) or a circle of knowledge which erased the individual. The dominant discursive formations have spread like volcanic ash, burning away maternal choice and creating a new hegemonic world order where breast IS best. Moreover, central to this new world order is the prominence of the baby and the absence of the mother. There may not be any clearer example of this erasure than the following declaration. According to the CDC, "2011 was a blessed year: 79 percent of newborns *started* (emphasis added) to breastfeed" (Breastfeeding Report Card, 2014, p. 2)! This statement begs the questions, how can a helpless and totally dependent newborn *start* to breastfeed without someone doing it for him/her? Moreover, whose breast is it and who's doing the feeding? Or most bluntly, where is the mom? In other words, by positioning the baby as the subject in the sentence, the true subject (the mother) is erased. This statement is just one example of the impact of the medi-institutionalized gaze contained in large part in the various pro-breastfeeding governmental, medical, and public health initiatives. Since "it is in discourse that power and knowledge are joined together" (Foucault, 1990, p. 100), we assert that the discourses of these documents and policies have created a breast-is-best discursive formation that is like a tight knot of surveillance and punishment for new mothers. Moreover, these initiatives and their corresponding discourses have enacted violence upon the female body as her breasts are ripped from it.

In this chapter we will review five such documents which have had a profound impact on creating the restrictive breast-is-best discursive formation and the maternal hegemonic world in which we currently live. These documents are as follows: 1.) The International Code of Marketing of Breast-milk Substitutes (The Code); 2.) Innocenti Declaration on the Protection, Promotion, and Support of Breastfeeding (The Declaration); 3.) The Baby-Friendly Hospital Initiative (BFHI); 4.) HHS Blueprint for Action on Breastfeeding (The Blueprint); and 5.) the Surgeon General's Call to Action to Support Breastfeeding (Call to Action).

DISCOURSE FIELDS AS IMPORTANT BACKDROP

Before reviewing the documents, it is important to remember that discursive formations are formed by numerous texts, objects, and statements (all broadly defined) that coalesce around a certain topic during a specific period in time, creating a particular knowledge about that topic. In our case, the knowledge/power is the breast-is-best discursive formation. In addition to the texts that we will review in this chapter, we need to remain cognizant of the times in which they were being created. Thus, the eras that we reviewed in chapter 2, and the corresponding discourses regarding social policy, political activity, conservatism, and feminist advocacy are integral to the construction of the breast-is-best paradigm. In addition, subsequent chapters examining discourses related to race, class, and resistance are all a part of the macro knowledge system as well.

As we discussed in chapter 2, there have been several different times in U.S. history that have been less female-friendly. The rise in conservatism years, during the Reagan (1980–1988) and George H. W. Bush (1988–1992) presidential years, along with the compassionate conservatism era of the George W. Bush (2000–2008) are certainly three of these time periods. Concomitantly, four of the five significant pro-breastfeeding policy documents were produced during this era of conservatism (see Table 3.1). Douglas and Michaels (2004) remind us that "the right wing of the Republican party—which controlled the White House from 1980 to 1992, [were] crucial years in the evolution of motherhood-hated the women's movement" (p. 10).

The 2011 Surgeon General's Call to Action to Support Breastfeeding is the only policy disseminated during the Obama presidency, which can be considered a more liberal, female friendly time. With that said, however, we will argue in this chapter that the more conservative governmental and medical authorities constructing the discourse have been far more powerful in controlling the narrative than their more liberal counterparts. Health professionals, Wright and Schanler concur when they stated in 2001 that "only of late have health professionals become involved in the promotion of breastfeeding as a return to traditional values and the 'natural' vs. the 'artificial' way to feed infants" (p. 421S). As the cacophony of these pro-natural, medical, and institutional discourses have grown louder so too have the binds of hegemonic mothering tightened significantly

Table 3.1. A Time Table of the Significant Pro-Breastfeeding Publications

Discourse Field	*Year Published*	*Document Name*
Our Body, Ourselves', or the Government's? (1970s–1980s)	1981	*The International Code of Marketing of Breast-milk Substitutes*
The Year of the Woman vs. the Moral Majority (1990s–2000s)	1990	*Innocenti Declaration on the Protection, Promotion, and Support of Breastfeeding*
The Year of the Woman vs. the Moral Majority (1990s–2000s)	1991	*The Baby-Friendly Hospital Initiative*
The Year of the Woman vs. the Moral Majority (1990s–2000s)	2000	*HHS Blueprint for Action on Breastfeeding*
Good Mothers Breastfeed; Bad Ones Do Not (2010s–2020s)	2011	*Surgeon General's Call to Action to Support Breastfeeding*

with the production of and abidance by the policies set forth in these significant documents. We argue that these documents, while created long ago, have had a tremendous impact on women's lives and are representative of the "guise of modern and enlightened 'gender aware' forms of govermentality" that discipline women in the twenty-first century (McRobbie, 2009, p. 2).

1981: THE INTERNATIONAL CODE OF MARKETING OF BREAST-MILK SUBSTITUTES

As the reader will recall, the *Our Body, Ourselves', or the Government's* discourse field of the 1970s and 1980s represented a tumultuous time of fighting for women's rights to their own bodies, their own paycheck, their own independence, on one hand, or for the need for women to return to their more traditional roles of wife and mother and to remain at home on the other. As women were becoming less tethered to the home, organizations such as the LLLI were arguing for the benefits of breastfeeding, which tied women to their babies, and, in turn, to their homes. It was also during this time that the Nestle case (see chapter 2 for more review) prompted an international effort to restrict marketing of formula in less-developed countries. In many ways, it became the tipping point for a groundswell of international interest during the latter part of the 1970s in improving the health of babies and young children among governments, scientists, nongovernmental organizations, manufacturers of infant formula, and professional organizations.

There was particular concern about the charges related to thousands of Third World babies dying of malnutrition and disease due to improper or unsanitary formula and baby food preparation.

As a result of this momentum, the World Health Organization (WHO) and the United Nations Children's Fund (UNICEF) convened a meeting in Geneva Switzerland in 1979 (International Code, 1981), which was attended by 150 representatives from WHO and UNICEF. Attendees agreed to the recommendation that "'there should be an international code of marketing of infant formula and other products used as breast-milk substitutes,' requesting the Director-General to prepare such a code 'in close consultation with Member States and with all other parties concerned'" (International Code, 1981, p. 5). After several drafts and subsequent resolutions, WHO adopted *The International Code of Marketing of Breast-milk Substitutes* (hereafter referred to as The Code). The Code is non-binding, but WHO member organizations were and have been urged to "translate it into national law and regulations" (Vandervort, 1981).

The United States was one of the three counties who did not support the resolution. According to the *Washington Post*, Gerald B. Helman, U.S. ambassador to the United Nations, told delegates after the vote, "We have serious concerns about this organization's involvement in commercial code and this is a central basis for our inability to support this code." He was referring primarily to Article 5 of The Code which states, "there shall be no advertising or other form of promotion to the general public of products within the scope of this code."

> Helman said the code's restrictions on the advertising of breast milk substitutes "cause serious legal and constitutional problems for the United States." The Reagan administration has indicated it believes such restrictions would be in violation of the First Amendment to the U.S. Constitution.
>
> He added that the U.S. government's rejection of the code did not imply a rejection of breast-feeding. "We strongly support efforts to promote and protect breast-feeding as the ideal form of infant nutrition," Helman stated. "Our own bilateral assistance programs encompassing education, training and dissemination of information in the promotion of breast-feeding and the improvement of infant and maternal nutrition attest to this commitment." (Vandervort, 1981)

In addition to the Reagan administration's concerns over free speech rights, one can postulate that their conservative beliefs in small government and big business with few regulations may have also impacted their decision to not adopt The Code. In so doing, it prioritized corporate rights and profitability over monitoring of infant formula. Interestingly, things have not changed much since the initial passing of The Code. The U.S. government still has taken no action to incorporate The Code into our laws. It supports a hands-off approach to governmental control of *corporations* but, as we will see, it does support a quasi-governmental control of *women's bodies*. In the United States, and arguably throughout Western civilization, gender equality is tied to individuality and economic purchasing power (McRobbie, 2009)—bedrocks of the patriarchal order that supports capitalism and classically liberal conservatism. This allows governmental actions (or inactions), like failing to accept The Code, to masquerade as empowering via capitalist ideology, while at the same time, controlling women's bodies. So, even though it has no legal authority in the United States, The Code has had a significant impact on other pro-breastfeeding initiatives and the current breast-is-best world in which we inhabit. Thus, it is worthy of our attention.

An archaeological dig into The Code's language reveals a privileging of the governmental and medical while infantilizing or erasing the mother. First, The Code's aim (Article 1) is to *protect and promote breastfeeding* by way of controlling the information disseminated and marketed about *breast-milk substitutes*. What passage and adoption of The Code meant for the women in developing countries is that infant feeding became a governmentally controlled behavior. Rather than being focused more on promoting the benefits of breastfeeding, the words of The Code implored governments to "protect" a maternal act from certain entities and individuals who were threatening to take it away. By putting serious restrictions on the information mothers receive about formula, the governments could be more certain that mothers will "choose" breastfeeding (see Table 3.2 for a summary of The Code with the most restrictive language highlighted). From a rhetorical perspective, The Code both empowers and limits, via language, at once bringing possibility to life, and restricting it (Hart, 1997).

Article 1: Aim

- The Code aims to protect and promote breastfeeding by ensuring appropriate use of breast-milk substitutes, when these are necessary, on the basis of adequate information and through appropriate marketing and distribution

Article 5: The general public and mothers

- No advertising or other forms of promotion to the general public of products within the scope of The Code
- No free samples of products within the scope of The Code provided to pregnant women, mothers, or members of their families
- No advertising, giving of samples, or other promotional strategies (e.g., special displays, discount coupons, special sales, etc.) to induce sales directly to the consumer
- No gifts of articles or utensils given to pregnant women, mothers, infants, or young children that may promote the use of breast-milk substitutes or bottle feeding
- No direct or indirect contact "of any kind" between marketing personnel and pregnant women or mothers of infants and young children

Article 7: Health workers

- Health workers should encourage and protect breastfeeding
- Information provided by manufacturers/distributors to health workers should be restricted to scientific facts; Information should not imply that bottle feeding is equal to or superior to breastfeeding
- Manufacturers/distributors should not offer nor should health care workers accept a financial or material inducement to promote products covered in The Code
- **No samples, equipment, or utensils should be provided to health care workers nor should health care workers give samples of formula to pregnant women, mothers, or members of their families**

Article 9: Labeling

- Labels should provide necessary information for appropriate use and should not discourage breastfeeding
- Labels on each container of formula **should not have pictures or text which idealizes formula** and should be clear, conspicuous, readable, and understandable and include the following:
    - the words "Important Notice" or their equivalent;
    - a statement of the superiority of breastfeeding; the terms "humanized," "materialized," or similar terms should not be used;
    - a statement that the product should be used only on the advice of a health worker as to the need for its use and the proper method of use

Table 3.2: Relevant Sections of the International Code of Marketing of Breast-milk Substitutes with restrictive language highlighted. Adapted from the International Code of Marketing of Breast-milk Substitutes (1981). Geneva, Switzerland: World Health Organization.

The governments who passed The Code were restricting mothers' rights to information and the ability to make their own independent, informed decisions on how to feed their baby. In essence, these governments were patronizing and infantilizing mothers by deciding for them what is best, like a parent would a child. Specifically, The Code limits mothers' agency by

- Allowing them to know only the benefits of breastfeeding and the negative impact of formula feeding.
- Informing them only of the costs and health hazards of formula.
- Disallowing them to receive any gifts or free samples of breast-milk substitutes, such as formula, or utensils that may promote bottle-feeding, such as pacifiers.
- Demeaning women's intelligence by restricting how formula is labeled.

So began the governmentalization and institutionalization of breastfeeding and the creation of the monitoring gaze. With the development of policies such as The Code, a creation of a structure allowed governments the capacity to observe the maternal body. As noted by Foucault (1994), "what was fundamentally invisible is suddenly offered to the brightness of the gaze" (p. 195).

The Code, while not officially passed in the United States, has had an enormous impact on all mothers and, as we'll see later, even medical facilities in the United States. It institutionalized and medicalized a "natural act" like breastfeeding, stripping mothers of the right to access all information they need to make decisions that are right for them and their families. The Code, and the governments that have enacted it, are determining for mothers what they should know and receive. Sadly, the impact of the gaze created by The Code was just the beginning.

1990: INNOCENTI DECLARATION ON THE PROTECTION, PROMOTION, AND SUPPORT OF BREASTFEEDING

As we have discussed, the 1980s was a period when we witnessed the rise of conservatism, the new right, the Cold War, and Reaganomics. It is also when The Code was voted on and began to influence global breastfeeding policy. While it is unlikely that a clear cause-and-effect relationship exists between The Code and rates of breastfeeding, it is clear that global governmental and public health interventions were driving the narrative and correspondingly, breastfeeding initiation did increase from its low in the 1970s to the mid 50th percentile in the 1980s.

However, initiation rates began to dip again in the latter part of the 1980s. To contextualize that change, we can look to several cultural, political, and governmental happenings during what we have labeled as the *Year of the Woman vs. the Moral Majority* discourse field (chapter 2). Briefly, George H. W. Bush, Reagan's vice president, won the presidency in 1988, continuing many of the Reagan era conservative values and policies. The United States experienced another economic recession from 1990–1991, which some say could be traced back to Black Monday in 1987, a worldwide drop in stocks (Karlgaard, 2010).

The late 1980s and early 1990s saw a decrease in men's participation in the workforce and median earnings but an increase in women's participation (U.S. Census Bureau, 2010). Women's-to-men's median earnings ratio also bumped up during this time period and women with a bachelor's degree or more (ages 25–29) surpassed those of men in the early 1990s.

As women were making significant progress with regard to pay equity, degree completion, and workforce participation, they also were freer to end dissatisfying and, perhaps even violent, marriages. They were also having fewer children and getting married later or never marrying at all. For example, from 1975 and 1990, the percentage of women never married declined from 63 percent to 38 percent (Norton & Miller, 1992). Just as we see women becoming more financially and relationally independent, we see additional and significant pro-breastfeeding initiatives, which placed pressure back on women to remain tethered to their children.

Notably, the *Innocenti Declaration on the Protection, Promotion, and Support of Breastfeeding* (The Declaration) was passed in 1990. In July of that year, policy makers from more than 30 countries gathered in Florence, Italy, and created The Declaration in an attempt to reverse declining breastfeeding rates (1990–2005, 2005). It was later endorsed by WHO and UNICEF, and unlike The Code, was signed onto by the United States. According to Marta Santos Pais, the Director of the UNICEF Innocenti Research Centre (1990–2005, 2005), The Declaration "captured the commitment as well as the practical vision of those who gathered in Florence to launch breastfeeding onto a higher public plane" (p. xii).

A close read of The Declaration (see Table 3.3) reveals ways in which, similar to The Code, governments, NGO's, and medical organizations continued to drive the narrative, set the agenda, and control the social discourse surrounding women's abilities to decide for themselves how to feed their children. Phrases such as "governments should develop . . . ." and "national authorities are urged" provide support for this perspective. With them in charge, breastfeeding is "protected" from the formula/bottle feeding invaders (aka the manufacturers/distributors), medical providers whose professionalism and expertise demand they attend to individual needs of each mother and baby, and mothers whose intellect and morals are questionable—for they would surely choose formula if their government wasn't "protecting" breastfeeding.

The Declaration recognized that breastfeeding is a unique process that:
• Provides ideal nutrition for infants and contributes to their healthy growth and development
• Provides social and economic benefits to the family and the nation
• Provides most women with a sense of satisfaction when successfully carried out
 	
The Declaration declared that:
• all women should be enabled to practice exclusive breastfeeding and all infants should be fed exclusively on breastmilk from birth to 4–6 months of age.
  ◦ Thereafter, children should continue to be breastfed, while receiving appropriate and adequate complementary foods, for up to two years of age or beyond.
  ◦ This child-feeding ideal is to be achieved by creating an appropriate environment of awareness and support so that women can breastfeed in this manner.
• this goal requires the reinforcement of a "breastfeeding culture" and its vigorous defense against incursions of a "bottle-feeding culture."
  ◦ This requires commitment and advocacy for social mobilization, utilizing to the full the prestige and authority of acknowledged leaders of society in all walks of life.
• efforts made to increase women's confidence in their ability to breastfeed.
  ◦ Such empowerment involves the removal of constraints and influences that manipulate perceptions and behavior towards breastfeeding, often by subtle and indirect means.
  ◦ This requires sensitivity, continued vigilance, and a responsive and comprehensive communications strategy involving all media and addressed to all levels of society.
  ◦ Furthermore, obstacles to breastfeeding within the health system, the workplace, and the community must be eliminated.
• governments should develop national breastfeeding policies and set appropriate national targets for the 1990s.
• national authorities urged to integrate their breastfeeding policies into their overall health and development policies.

Table 3.3: A Partial Summary of the Innocenti Declaration on The Protection, Promotion and Support of Breastfeeding Data from *Innocenti Declaration on the Protection, Promotion, and Support of Breastfeeding* (1990). New York City: UNICEF.

With this type of language, The Declaration creates a tight feedback loop, reminding governments to continue to support The Code and other previously passed pro-breastfeeding initiatives. It continues to perpetuate the need to support the "'breastfeeding culture' by defending it from the 'incursions' of a 'bottle-feeding culture.'" This loop becomes closed from outside "interference" (e.g., "removal of constraints and influences" and "obstacles to breastfeeding" must be eliminated), thereby being allowed to perpetuate its own ideology.

We see mothers minimized, at best, and often erased from much of this edict. For example, the opening lines declare that breastfeeding is a unique process that provides ideal nutrition, reduces incidence of infectious diseases, and contributes to women's health. When women are mentioned, they are referenced in the last of four operational targets and are discursively positioned as passive agents needing to have their confidence in breastfeeding increased. As The Declaration declares, women's confidence is increased by *removing constraints and negative influences* about breastfeeding, *controlling the communication* they receive from media *and eliminating* (for them) *obstacles* to breastfeeding in the health system, the workplace, and the community. Accordingly, women's confidence is increased, not by being given agency and access to all information, but instead by being stripped of their autonomy. The Declaration also recognizes that breastfeeding is beneficial to the family AND THE NATION, while providing *most women with a sense of satisfaction when successfully carried out.* So, by subverting their own agenic control over their bodies, mothers are also able to carry out their patriotic duty by breastfeeding their infant and *most* of them should receive some sense of satisfaction for doing so. The Declaration (and others like it) further reinforces the medi-institutional gaze which provides constant surveillance and monitoring of *the breast* while dismembering it from the mother's body. The words become gospel and the breast becomes sacred. Mothers become the sacrificial lambs for their children!

1991: THE BABY-FRIENDLY HOSPITAL INITIATIVE (BFHI)

One of The Declaration's operational targets was to guarantee that every facility providing maternity services practice a set of steps to ensure breastfeeding success. A first step in that process was the creation by WHO and UNICEF of a document entitled "'Protecting, Promoting and Supporting Breast-feeding: The Special Role of Maternity Services.' This document outlined 'Ten Steps to Successful Breastfeeding'" (hereafter called The Steps) (1990–2005, 2005, p. 6). Close attention to the language of The Steps (see Table 3.4) underscores once again the absence of mothers in the instructions, the constraints on their autonomy, the myopic ideological approach to infant feeding, and the tight restrictions on health care staff.

Even with such restrictive, dogmatic ideology, The Steps have had tremendous impact on the perpetuation of the breast-is-best policy and practice worldwide, including the United States. It became the foundation for the establishment of the Baby-Friendly Hospital Initiative (BFHI), which was inaugurated by WHO and UNICEF in 1991. The BFHI is a worldwide program aimed at encouraging birthing facilities to follow The Steps and mothers to breastfeed their newborns (Baby-Friendly, 2016). There were three primary goals of BFHI:

- "Improve breastfeeding practices within maternity wards in the health system;

Table 3.4. Ten Steps to Successful Breastfeeding

Step Number	*Required Action*
1.	Have a written breastfeeding policy that is routinely communicated to all health care staff.
2.	Train all health care staff in skills necessary to implement this policy.
3.	Inform all pregnant women about the benefits and management of breastfeeding.
4.	Help mothers initiate breastfeeding within one half-hour of birth.
5.	Show mothers how to breastfeed and maintain lactation, even if they should be separated from their infants.
6.	Give newborn infants no food or drink other than breast-milk, unless medically indicated.
7.	Practice rooming-in—that is, allow mothers and infants to remain together 24 hours a day.
8.	Encourage breastfeeding on demand.
9.	Give no artificial teats or pacifiers (also called dummies or soothers) to breastfeeding infants.
10.	Foster the establishment of breastfeeding support groups and refer mothers to them on discharge from the hospital or clinic.

Source: Protecting and Supporting Breastfeeding: The Special Role of Maternity Services, a Joint WHO/UNICEF Statement Published by the World Health Organization (1989). Note: For 2018 revised 10 Steps see https://www.who.int/nutrition/bfhi/ten-steps/en/

- Educate all health workers who were trained in these facilities concerning the importance and basic skills of breastfeeding support; and
- Enforce within facilities the principles of the International Code of Marketing of Breast-milk Substitutes." (1990–2005, 2005)

As of 2016, more than 170 countries had begun implementation and more than 20,000 birth facilities worldwide had received official designation (Baby-Friendly, 2016). The first baby-friendly designated facility in the United States occurred in 1996 (Country experiences, 2017). Shortly thereafter, in 1997, Baby-Friendly, USA, a non-governmental, non-profit organization was created (Baby-Friendly, 2016) to serve as the accrediting body for BFHI implementation (Country experiences, 2017). According to Baby-Friendly, USA, Inc., as of June 2018, there were 528 BFHI approved hospitals and birthing centers across all 50 states, the District of Columbia, and Puerto Rico (The Baby-Friendly, n.d.). As accredited birthing facilities have increased, so too has the percentage of children born at BFHI hospitals. In 2016, for example, 12 percent of birthing facilities in the United States were BFHI approved, and nearly 20 percent of infants were born at these types of institutions (Country experiences, 2017).

Becoming Baby-Friendly

As noted earlier, Baby-Friendly USA oversees the conferral of BFHI designation to birthing facilities in the United States. As part and parcel of the process, facilities need to implement the 10 Steps, successfully complete an external evaluation, and comply with The Code—even though the United States has not legislatively implemented it (Country experiences, 2017). What is not apparent, however, in the label is that to earn baby-friendly designation the facility, its workers, and its mothers must ascribe to the breast-at-all costs dogma. Table 3.5 includes a partial summary of the guidelines and evaluation criteria hospitals need to implement in order to become baby-friendly.

Proponents have accredited the BFHI for getting breastfeeding on health policy agenda of countries across the world and for increasing exclusive breastfeeding "in many regions, even in the face of continued advertising of commercial infant foods and increasing HIV prevalence" (1990–2005, 2005, p. 7).

On the other hand, opponents argue that it has radicalized the breast-is-best phenomenon. The discursive development of BFH looks very similar to the birth of the clinic as outlined by Foucault (1994). There was a rather "sudden, restructuring" of how hospitals served pregnant women and their families. Foucault (1994) notes that

> For clinical experience to become possible as a form of knowledge, a reorganization of the hospital field, a new definition of the status of the patient in society, and the establishment of a certain relationship between public assistance and medical experience, between help and knowledge, become necessary: the patient has to be enveloped in a collective, homogeneous space. (p. 196)

The creation of the breastfeeding hospital meant that decisions were removed from women and their families and placed in the hands of institutional and medical professionals. The "knowing subject" shifted from the mother and to the organizations and medical systems (Foucault, 1995). These larger systems are thereby controlling the discourse and surveilling the moms (as well as the employees) (Foucault, 1994, 1995). Mothers at BFH are caught in a double system of observation—a gaze telling them that breastfeeding is natural and the best way to feed their babies as well as a gaze isolating them within a medical system with one specific ideology—BREAST IS BEST! While the BFHI has only continued to grow and surveil mothers in this way, the U.S. government created some of its own documents/initiatives which have only continued this process.

Step 1: Have a written breastfeeding policy that is routinely communicated to all health care staff.

- Breast milk should be the standard for infant feeding. All infants in the facility should be considered to be breastfeeding infants unless, after giving birth and being offered help to breastfeed, the mother has specifically stated that she has no plans to breastfeed.
- The Ten Steps to Successful Breastfeeding (Ten Steps) and a statement indicating the facility's adherence to the WHO International Code requirements related to the purchase and promotion of breast milk substitutes, bottles, nipples, pacifiers, and other infant feeding supplies should be prominently displayed in all areas that serve mothers, infants, and young children.

Step 2. Train all health care staff in the skills necessary to implement this policy.

- At minimum, all health care providers must have a true understanding of the benefit of exclusive breastfeeding, physiology of lactation, how their specific field of practice impacts lactation, and how to find out about safe medications for use during lactation.
- The facility should determine the amount and content of training required by staff in other units and roles by their anticipated workplace exposure to mothers and infants.
- Examples of training for staff outside of maternity include, but are not limited to:
    - Pharmacist—importance of exclusive breastfeeding, medications acceptable for breastfeeding
    - Anesthesiologist—importance of exclusive breastfeeding, importance of immediate skin-to-skin contact
    - Radiology—importance of exclusive breastfeeding, where to find out about safe medications for use during lactation, where to find appropriate information on use of radioisotopes during lactation
    - Housekeeping staff—importance of exclusive breastfeeding, practices that support breastfeeding, the facility's philosophy on infant nutrition, who to call when a mother needs help

Step 6: Give infants no food or drink other than breast milk, unless medically indicated.

- Exclusive breast milk feeding shall be the feeding method expected from birth to discharge.
- When a mother specifically states that she has no plans to breastfeed or requests that her breastfeeding infant be given a breast milk substitute, the health care staff should first explore the reasons for this request, address the concerns raised, and educate her about the possible consequences to the health of her infant and the success of breastfeeding. If the mother still requests a breast milk substitute, her request should be granted and the process and the informed decision should be documented.

Step 7: Practice rooming in—allow mothers and infants to remain together 24 hours a day.

Step 9: Give no pacifiers or artificial nipples to breastfeeding infants.

- Health care professionals, including nursery staff, should educate all breastfeeding mothers about how the use of bottles and artificial nipples may interfere with the development of optimal breastfeeding. When a mother requests that her breastfeeding infant be given a bottle, the health care staff should explore the reasons for this request, address the concerns raised, educate her on the possible consequences to the success of

Table 3.5: A Summary of The Guidelines and Evaluation Criteria for Hospital and Birthing Center Implementation of the U.S. Baby-Friendly Hospital Initiative (with critical text highlighted). Data from Baby-Friendly USA (2016). Guidelines and Evaluation Criteria for Facilities Seeking Baby-Friendly Designation. Albany, NY: Baby-Friendly USA, 2016.

breastfeeding, and discuss alternative methods for soothing and feeding her infant. If the mother still requests a bottle, the process of counseling and education and the informed decision of the mother should be documented.
In addition:
Compliance with the International Code of Marketing of Breast-milk Substitutes
• The facility will demonstrate its compliance with the International Code by refusing to accept supplies of breast milk substitutes and feeding supplies at no cost or below fair market cost, by protecting new parents from the influence of vendors of such items, by practicing in accordance with its vendor and ethics policies regarding appropriate interaction between vendors of such items and facility staff, and by educating staff members about the International Code and its role in ethical health care practices.

Table 3.5 Continued.

2000: HHS BLUEPRINT FOR ACTION ON BREASTFEEDING

In addition to signing The Declaration in 1990, the U.S. government became very involved from the mid-1980s to the early 1990s with numerous breastfeeding promotion activities, such as workshops, conferences, publications, legislation, policies, media campaigns, and research (HHS Blueprint, 2000). In 1984, for example, the Office of the Surgeon General held "the first workshop on breastfeeding and human lactation" (HHS Blueprint, 2000, p. 3). Concurrently, the U.S. Department of Health and Human Services developed Healthy People 2000 which was the first set of national targets for infant health concerning breastfeeding rates. The Healthy People 2000 objectives for breastfeeding were to increase breastfeeding initiation rates to 75 percent and to increase to 50 percent the proportion of babies breastfed at 6 months (HHS Blueprint, 2000). Despite monumental efforts, the 2000 goals were not met (HHS Blueprint, 2000).

However, not to be deterred and to help reach the Healthy People 2010 breastfeeding goals, Dr. David Satcher, the Assistant Secretary for Health and Surgeon General, requested additional governmental agencies and health care organizations help him develop The Blueprint for Action on Breastfeeding, which established "a comprehensive breastfeeding policy for the nation" (HHS Blueprint, 2000, p. 4). The Blueprint asserts that "infants should be exclusively breastfed during the first 4 to 6 months of life . . . , preferably for a full 6 months . . . . Ideally, breastfeeding should continue through the first year of life" (p. 19). It goes on to call on governmental agencies, health facilities, and many others to take up this *call to action,*

> Achieving an increase in the proportion of mothers who breastfeed their babies will require the collaboration of Federal agencies, State and local governments, communities, health professional organizations, advocacy groups, multidisciplinary scientists, industry, health insurers

> and the American people. The Blueprint for Action invites all interested stakeholders to forge partnerships for the promotion of breastfeeding. It is also designed to attract broad-based family, community, professional, corporate, and philanthropic participation in order to better focus the public's attention and to motivate actions at the individual and community levels. (p. 19)

The Blueprint's focus on the involvement of various stakeholders to increase the proportion of women who breastfeed is laudable. Yet, it isn't until after this long declaratory statement of purpose before they finally get to the mothers. The second paragraph of the Action statement starts with the following sentence, "Moreover, this Blueprint for Action is directed toward all women and cuts across all racial and ethnic populations, socio-economic classes, educational groups, and employment arrangements" (p. 19). The word "Moreover" is synonymous with other phrases like "a further matter," "in addition to," "what's more" as if the mothers were an additional thing to be considered instead of "fundamental," "central to," or a "key focus" to such calls to action.

Following the general statement of its purpose, The Blueprint recommends several steps be taken to achieve the breastfeeding objectives for the Healthy People 2010 initiative. These steps and associated objectives were in the health care system, workplace, family and community, and research. All oriented once again toward protecting, supporting, and promoting breastfeeding. The act is once again removed from the authentic actor—the mother. Mother's needs, wishes, and desires are subsumed to the agenic forces of the government. The act of breastfeeding is the holy grail.

With that said, there were several refreshing discursive positions in The Blueprint that marked a deviation from language used in past institution edicts. For instance, it noted the racial and ethnic disparities in breastfeeding rates and called for more research that "identified the social, cultural, economic, and psychological factors that influence infant feeding behaviors, especially among African American and other minority and ethnic groups" (p. 20). Additionally, verbs such as "encourage," "facilitate," "develop," "compare," and "conduct" were used throughout the recommended action steps instead of the words should/should not, requires, may not, no (samples, advertising, information, etc.), and no idealizing that permeate The Code and The Declaration. Discursive space is opened up by these more interactive, dialogic verbs, thereby creating more agenic maternal control.

Finally, of the significant pro-breastfeeding initiatives and corresponding documents we have discussed herein, The Blueprint (2000) is the first one to include cautionary tales about how breast milk can be affected by such things as environmental toxins, drugs, and diseases. It is unique in its willingness to acknowledge that not all breast milk is safe—something virtually left unsaid in The Code and The Declaration. So, with The Blueprint, we see some shifting in the medi-institutionalized gaze. Its focus remains on the breast and the act of breastfeeding, but the mothers' subjection is lessoned.

2011: SURGEON GENERAL'S CALL TO ACTION TO SUPPORT BREASTFEEDING

In recognition of the 10th anniversary of the *HHS Blueprint for Action on Breastfeeding,* U.S. Surgeon General Regina M. Benjamin issued *The 2011 Surgeon General's Call to Action to Support Breastfeeding* (2011) recognizing the need for continued public support for breastfeeding mothers. The 90+ page report includes information on the importance of breastfeeding, rates of disparity, barriers to breastfeeding, breastfeeding from the public health perspective, and a call to action.

Even though this is one more governmental document dictating how mothers should behave, its tone is very different from others. Unlike The Code, The Declaration, and even The Blueprint which prioritized protecting, promoting, and supporting breastfeeding, the Call to Action is different. We must be mindful that the Call to Action was created during the Obama administration which had many more women in high positions of power and was thought to be more female-centric (see chapter 2 for discussion of Good Mothers Breastfeed; Bad Ones Do Not discourse field). According to Surgeon General Benjamin, she

> issued this *Call to Action* because the time has come to set forth the important roles and responsibilities of clinicians, employers, communities, researchers, and government leaders and to urge us all to take on a commitment to enable mothers to meet their personal goals for breastfeeding. Mothers are acutely aware of and devoted to their responsibilities when it comes to feeding their children, but the responsibilities of others must be identified so that all mother can obtain the information, help, and support they deserve when they breastfeed these infants. (p. v)

Although the focus is still on the exclusivity of breastfeeding, the fact that mothers' needs have received some higher order of attention cannot be under-appreciated. There are 20 action steps and associated implementation strategies (categorized within 6 thematic areas) in the Call to Action (see Table 3.6). The very first theme is "Mothers and their Families" and the first action step is "Give mothers the support they need to breastfeed their babies" (p. 38)! Health care professionals are empowered to provide women with "accurate and complete information on infant feeding as a part of routine prenatal care, but if not provided, mothers have the right to ask for it. Mothers can obtain this information from their clinicians to ensure they have the knowledge they need to make the decision about infant feeding that is best for them" (Call to Action, 2011). There is also

Table 3.6. Actions to Improve Breastfeeding

Mothers and Their Families:

Action 1: Give mothers the support they need to breastfeed their babies.

Action 2: Develop programs to educate fathers and grandmothers about breastfeeding.

Communities:

Action 3: Strengthen programs that provide mother-to-mother support and peer counseling.

Action 4: Use community-based organizations to promote and support breastfeeding.

Action 5: Create a national campaign to promote breastfeeding.

Action 6: Ensure that the marketing of infant formula is conducted in a way that minimizes its negative impacts of exclusive breastfeeding.

Health Care:

Action 7: Ensure that maternity care practices throughout the United States are fully supportive of breastfeeding.

Action 8: Develop systems to guarantee continuity of skilled support for lactation between hospitals and health care settings in the community.

Action 9: Provide education and training in breastfeeding for all health professionals who care for women and children.

Action 10: Include basic support for breastfeeding as a standard of care for midwives, obstetricians, family physicians, nurse practitioners, and pediatricians.

Action 11: Ensure access to services provided by Internal Board Certified Lactation Consultants.

Action 12: Identify and address obstacles to greater availability of safe banked donor milk for fragile infants.

Employment:

Action 13: Work toward establishing paid maternity leave for all employed mothers.

Action 14: Ensure that employers establish and maintain comprehensive, high-quality lactation support programs for their employees.

Action 15: Expand the use of programs in the workplace that allow lactating mothers to have direct access to their babies.

Action 16: Ensure that all child care providers accommodate the needs of breastfeeding mothers and infants.

Research and Surveillance:

Action 17: Increase funding of high-quality research on breastfeeding.

Action 18: Strengthen existing capacity and develop future capacity for conducting research on breastfeeding.

Action 19: Develop a national monitoring system to improve the tracking of breastfeeding rates as well as the policies and environmental factors that affect breastfeeding.

Public Health Infrastructure:

Action 20: Improve national leadership on the promotion and support of breastfeeding.

Source: The Surgeon General's call to action to support breastfeeding (2011). Washington, DC: U.S. Department of Health and Human Services. Office of the Surgeon General.

more of a focus on structures that are necessary for all mothers to breastfeed should they so desire. Yet, taking a step back, we can still see the Call to Action's focus on *breastfeeding*. The mothers remain the docile body, which can "be subjected, used, transformed, and improved" (Foucault, 1995, p. 136)—and monitored.

2019 AND BEYOND

> The state that I depict will have a simple, reliable, easily controlled administration. It will resemble those huge machines, which by quite uncomplicated means produce great effects; the strength of the state will spring from its own strength, its prosperity from its own prosperity. Time, which destroys all, will increase its power. (Foucault, 1995, p. 168)

Like Foucault's conception of state, the disjointed but yet interconnected administrative pro-breastfeeding initiatives and the huge machinery that they have created has produced great effects. Over time, as demonstrated in the documents reviewed herein, we have seen the power of the medicalization and institutionalization of a "natural" feminine bodily act become stronger and stronger. The medi-institutionalized gaze created, supported, and perpetuated in these grand initiatives and documents has made the female body an object that can be manipulated, pulled apart, and used for financial gain. Large global and national organizations have used her body, our bodies, as a means of perpetuating their own raison d-etra and creating a new "political anatomy" (Foucault, 1995). Holding power over the now docile, female body, affords them the ability to operate as they wish and to discipline us. All of these documents include some sort of call for action, calls for marketing controls of formula, for protecting breastfeeding, and creating medical facilities that are judged by their baby-friendliness. Hospitals are spending thousands of dollars to become baby-friendly because what mom wouldn't want to deliver their baby at such a place. For example, one analysis showed that in 2013 it would cost hospitals with more than 500 births per year, approximately $322,000 to go through the accreditation process to be designated "a baby-friendly hospital" (Delli Fraine, Langabeer II, Delgado, Williams, & Gong, 2013).

Moreover, as part of the big machinery, the baby-friendly hospitals have had to create a discourse field that demands hospitals monitor breastfeeding rates, ascribe to the breast-is-the only-option ideology, and require employees take an oath to advocate that ideal and pledge to support only breastfeeding. There is a type of force within this discourse field. It's one of those instances when the choice not to conform becomes unthinkable. What hospital wouldn't want to become baby-friendly? What mom would want to deliver her baby at a non-baby-friendly hospital. The pressure to comply has passed the stage of optional but instead has become obligatory. Yet, to be fair, BFH have been allowed to be created because of all the medical, social, political, and institutional discourses working together in the creation of the breast-is-best discursive formation. This discourse has turned mothers into patients and breastfeeding into a medical intervention by which the state (broadly defined) can exert authority.

As we bring this chapter to a close, we invite you to envision a new world order with us—one that can challenge the dual gendered notion of femininity that only offers freedom through purchasing power and not wholesale change of the social structures that discipline women and our bodies (see McRobbie, 2009). Dare we imagine this radical world of Mother-Friendly Hospitals? One in which facilities, workers, and a social world respects women enough to give them all of the facts surrounding infant feeding choices? That allow marketing of all baby-related materials as appropriate, so women can see what options exist? That teach women about the options, advantages, and disadvantages of different types of formulas, bottles, nipples, and pacifiers? That share with women the benefits and costs of breastfeeding—alongside those of formula? That give mothers access to free samples, so they can try before they buy? That recognizes that all mothers, babies, and families benefit from "rooming in" and skin-to-skin contact regardless of feeding method?

We must push back against the medi-institutional-governmentalized gaze that is partly the result of the documents reviewed herein and other policy initiatives too many to mention. We must ask important questions such as why is there a need to control and surveil mothers? Why is there a need to "protect" breastfeeding by keeping information away from women? We strongly believe that, with more freedom and information, many mothers can take possession once again of their bodies and their free will. Many will still choose the breast; Others will not. There is enough evidence to show that both options—at least in the United States—are just fine.

FOUR

Disciplining the Maternal Body

Discourses for Expecting Moms

As we have discussed, the 1980s was an era when *Our Body, Ourselves', or the Government's?* field of discourse subjected women's bodies to more surveillance and discipline in reaction to the freedoms gained during the 1960s and 1970s. The era also was a time when governmental agencies and cultural organizations, such as LLLI, were creating policies and practices to increase breastfeeding rates with great success. The medi-institutional gaze, or in other words, the objectification, surveillance, and discipline of women/mothers, began to develop during this time period as a result of numerous socio-political movements such as the rise in conservatism, the Nestle scandal which prompted strict formula regulations, the creation of the International Code of Marketing of Breast-milk Substitutes, and the Surgeon General's Healthy People Objectives for 1990 which, among other health initiatives, focused on increasing breastfeeding rates.

At the same time—and perhaps in response to the increased attention on women's pregnant and feeding bodies—pregnancy and parenting books began to top best-selling lists. For instance, since its release in 1984, *What to Expect When You're Expecting* has sold more than 17 million copies worldwide (Pederson & Effron, 2012). As the leader in sales for the "pregnancy and childbirth" genre, "*What to Expect*" is marketed as "the bible for moms-to-be and their families" (Pederson & Effron, 2012). With such success, additional books flooded the market. As we write this book, the top selling pregnancy and childbirth books are: *The Mayo Clinic's Guide to a Healthy Pregnancy* and *Pregnancy; The Complete Guide to Everything You Need to Know About a Healthy Pregnancy That Fits Your Lifestyle;* and *Healing Your Body After Childbirth* (Amazon.com, Childbirth and Pregnancy).

Together, these books, their sequels (*What to Expect in the First Year of Life*), and their numerous counterparts make up the pregnancy and childbirth genre, which can be viewed as a discursive/rhetorical genre, or a grouping of persuasive texts that seek to provide helpful advice for new moms/parents. At the same time, this genre promotes a particular perspective of pregnancy and infant care that limits ways of understanding both. It cannot be ignored that these books were becoming popular at the same time as the medi-institutional, pro-breastfeeding gaze was surveilling and disciplining mothers, and that as this gaze intensified its focus on women, more books offering similar advice filled bookstore shelves and online suggestion feeds. As we will argue in this chapter, these books became another way of disciplining the maternal body by rhetorically persuading and shaping pro-breastfeeding practices.

As part of a larger discourse of femininity, these books aid in the creation of a single form of motherhood—a hegemonic stronghold that reverberates throughout maternal discourses. In relationship to the same white, heteronormative suppositions found in the breastfeeding initiatives discussed throughout the book, the discourses of the pregnancy and childbirth genre create a white, virtuous, quasi-religious maternal archetype that acts as an "epistemic individual, an individual whose social position illuminates the gendered dynamics at work in media morality narratives that characterize senses of hegemonic femininity" (Favre, 2015, p. 627). This chapter explores how the idea of "mother" becomes a "maternal form of moral authority based on a particular gendered, raced, and classed position" (Favre, 2015, p. 627). We begin this exploration by discussing how generic analysis reveals the "rules" of a particular genre and how this intersects with discursive analysis as discussed in chapter 2. We then further examine the concept of hegemonic motherhood and its relationship with breastfeeding. We conclude this chapter with an analysis of the top selling pregnancy and childbirth books.

DISCURSIVE FORMATION AND GENERIC RHETORICAL CRITICISM

As readers may recall, we have defined discursive formations as a rule set that "governs the way that a topic can be meaningfully talked about and reasoned about. It also influences how ideas are put into practice and used to regulate the conduct of others" (Hall, 2001, p. 72). We argue that the pregnancy and childbirth book genre, which is dedicated to disseminating information, functions as a set of discursive formations and is generic in that these books rely on a limited number of options, or events. That is to say, while there are an infinite number of birthing and child feeding experiences, and any number of ways "to do" both, a complex dynamic of social and biological discursive formations "narrow" the process into the singular, often biological reality of mothering. In the case of giving birth, Rodgers (2015) explains:

> Various interest groups including feminist movements, women's health movements and home-birth campaigners have vigorously campaigned for a return to a natural model of pregnancy and childbirth. It can be argued that as a result of these ideological conflicts, women have a large number of choices with regard to childbirth. . . . However, Edwards (2004) describes the availability of such choices as largely constrained by social factors that "the intersection between ideology and resources results in a predetermined, medically oriented menu over which women have limited control to define or change" (p. 2–3). The discourses of pregnancy and childbirth of the late 20th century and early 21st century shaped by these socio-cultural factors are complex and reflect the ideological conflicts between medical and natural models of pregnancy and childbirth. (p. 40)

In the case of child feeding, the practice of feeding is reduced to a singular act, while the reality of womanhood and motherhood are variably complex:

> The medical discussion of the physiological aspects of breastfeeding articulates conflicting ideological views of women and their place in society, demonstrating how medicine reflects and contributes to a cultural context that is ambivalent about women's changing roles and the transformation of their practices as mothers. (Hausman, 2000, p. 271)

Discursive formations both create and restrict social reality by policing social norms and dictating behavior. In this case, they are enacting dual gendered realities by assuming women's autonomy, and at the same time requiring them to be *all woman* (McRobbie, 2009). Limiting the scope of social reality translates into limited expectations of social actors. The result is reflective of Perelman and Olbrechts-Tyteca's (1969) notion of the universal audience, where rhetors (authors) are incarnations of the audience. This is to say that in recognizing their audience's needs, desires, values, and expectations, author-ities[1] rearticulate these limited social expectations in the form of persuasive appeals. In terms of our topic, most of us "know" about pregnancy and childbirth well before we've ever experienced it. Even though few of us experience pregnancy in the same way, we have expectations of what we should expect to know. Childhood and pregnancy books limit information in order to meet the *a priori* expectations of readers. Analyzing those limitations requires the critic to employ generic criticism.

Genre and Discourse

According to Hart (1997), "a genre is a class of messages having important structural and content similarities and which, as a class, creates special expectations in listeners" (p. 122). As critics, we use these classes of rhetoric to unmask value systems because, as Hart (1997) explains, "generic patterns reveal societal truths" (p. 122). "The generic critic examines message patterns in order to comment on the universal as manifested in the particular" (Hart, 1997, p. 122). Genres are also organizing tools. They are conservative pieces of rhetoric that "keep things in place" (Hart, 1997, p. 123). Because generic analysis places equal emphasis on what is said, as well as what is left out of a text, this type of criticism also allows critics to demonstrate the power and motivation that guides both the presence and absence of particular concepts.

Formal analysis of texts provides critics with additional insight into the notion of presence and absence. "The centrality of structure to content is best seen when structure is missing or misappropriated" (the presence of absence) (Hart, 1997, p. 110). Formal analysis examines the form and structure of texts to take into account what is said and when, how much or how little is said, and where it is said, to reveal the emphasis placed on certain actions in relation to others (Hart, 1997). Criticism of syntax and imagery provides additional support, here. Primary structures and secondary structures reveal "truths" and preferences. Imagery and style force us to ask what purpose things like wording serve, and like generic criticism, can reveal the author's motives (Burke, 1969). For this analysis, we are drawing on multiple tools from the rhetorical critic's toolbox because:

> approaching the same message from numerous perspectives builds in safeguards against foolishness. To appreciate the subtlety of language, one must get beyond impressionism by categorizing and counting. . . . Language is wonderful. . . . All of us love it. But like any lover, it must not be taken for granted. The good stylistic critic never does. (Hart, 1997, p. 133)

From a discursive standpoint, this analysis allows us to illuminate "the often opaque connections between language and other aspects of society and culture" (Fairclough, 1996, p. 286). We can see how the rhetoric operationalized, while concomitantly revealing the limitations placed on discourses through discursive policing. As meanings change, in terms of Foucault and genealogy, so to do the possibilities.

Analyzing Generic Rhetoric through Structure and Form

Structure is "the appointment and sequencing of message elements. Structural decisions are decisions about which ideas should be given what amount of attention and how ideas should be arranged for maximum impact" (Hart, 1997, p. 107). We can think of this as the rhetorical tool of "elimination sequence" or "a solution-oriented approach in which all but one remedy is successively eliminated by the speaker" (Hart, 1997, p. 107). Form is "the patterns of meaning listeners generate when they take in a message" (Hart, 1997, p. 108). While form is harder to analyze textually, a speaker's aspirations of formation can be discerned from textual analysis. Hart (1997) tells the critic to analyze "which points are *emphasized* and which are given short shift . . . do these decisions expose the persuasive obstacle being faced (italics original)" (p. 118)?

Since few real-life messages follow precise rules, form is difficult to ascertain, but good communicators will provide listeners with "organizational help" (Hart, 1997, p. 111). Structural analysis examines the following: 1) "message design (the use of standard structural devices)"; 2) "message emphasis (the comparative treatment of individual ideas)"; 3) "message density (the depth of coverage of individual ideas)"; and 4) "message pacing (the distribution of ideas through time)" (Hart, 1997, p. 111).

From a contextual standpoint, the critic is asking, "does an idea's context give it special importance or attractiveness? Do the statements made just before or just after an idea make it less likely or more likely that that idea will be received well (understood and accepted)" (Hart, 1997, p. 116). In addition, a critic wants to know, "how much time is spent on the introduction of *novel* information? How much time is spent recasting the familiar? Does this known/unknown ratio reveal anything important about the rhetorical situation" (Hart, 1997, p. 118)?

Rhetorical critics should take into account which ideas dominate the text and how they are articulated (message density) (Hart, 1997). Taking care to note how certain ideas are proffered over others reveals the *a priori* attitudes and beliefs with which the author assumes the audience engages the text. Are these ideas presented as common sense? Does the author assume everyone is in agreement? Or, does the author try to dissuade readers from a particular action, belief, or idea? If there are controversial topics, when are they presented? Why? Does the arrangement of ideas lead a reader to certain conclusions? Each of these questions fall to the rhetorical critic (Hart, 1997). At a micro level, generic, formal, and structural analyses allow critics to unmask a message's underlying motives. At a macro level, it can reveal a society's values and beliefs—the taken for granted norms that organize everyday life.

HEGEMONIC MOTHERHOOD ARTICULATED WITHIN CHILDBIRTH AND PARENTING BOOKS

In her historical account of parenting books, Hulbert (2003) highlights what she (and as her book demonstrates, many others) considers to be the uniquely American fixation on rearing children . . . perfectly. Hulbert's work is an examination of a centuries worth of parenting books which ultimately demonstrates that even though the act of sustaining life remains constant for every generation of parents (i.e., we want to keep them alive), the enactment of sustaining life changes drastically in conjunction with drastic cultural changes. For example, if we look to the timelines presented in chapter 2, we see that the 1950s and 1960s were a period where technological advancements provided women with more options, but those options were met with resistance. Hulbert (2003) notes that parenting books of the same time period:

> sounded more worried and at odds then ever, their audience of women challenging the demands and constrictions of that "vocation of motherhood." America's families, although they had, of course never been homogenous, had never been so diverse—or seemed so precarious. There was hardly time for hesitancy: the harried working parent and the "hurried child" had become the type of the times. (p. 6)

Hulbert's work demonstrates that pregnancy and childbirth books—as a body of work—often fail to provide the calm and consistency they advocate. Rather, they are reactionary texts that reflect the social exigencies they exist within. "The truth is that both the advocates of more authority for parents, and the proponents of greater intimacy with children have betrayed their fair share of ambivalence about their own theories and advice" (Hulbert, 2003, p. 7). So perhaps rather than view these books as gospel and/or technological truths, we should view them as pieces of work existing within specific discursive frameworks. As evidenced with our timelines in chapter 2, Hulbert's examination of parenting books reveals that early twentieth century experts touted science as a means of rearing new, previously unseen generations of advanced citizens. However, at just about the same time those scientific advancements that helped us understand medicine, vaccinations, and brain activity, also led to advancements in women's health and control over reproduction, the books took an about turn. The "unbiased experts" reverted to natural methods of child rearing, using evidence of stressed and lonely children as proof that science had led us astray.

Acting as author-ities over the experience of birthing and breastfeeding, the authors of each book analyzed in this section have various qualifications when it comes to breastfeeding and infant care. *The Mayo Clinic Guide to a Health Pregnancy* (2018) is written by Myra J. Wick, MD, PhD, a "specialist in the Department of Obstetrics and Gynecology and the Department of Clinical Genomics at Mayo Clinic" (Wick, 2018, [Kindle version, location 47]). Her experience as a doctor, professor, and mother lends her a certain amount of credibility, specifically in terms of pregnancy's biological components. The *Guide's* follow up, *The Mayo Clinic's Guide to a Healthy First Year* (2018), is cleverly touted as a book written by "Doctors who are parents too!" and performs similarly in terms of form and content. These books' focus on balanced medical advice sets them apart from the arguably more popular, "pop-culture" books like *What to Expect When You're Expecting* (2012), *What to Expect in the First Year,* and

Pregnancy: The Complete Guide to Everything You Need to Know About a Healthy Pregnancy That Fits Your Lifestyle and *Healing Your Body After Childbirth*. These latter examples are not written by medical professionals, but at least in the case of *Expecting* (and less so in "*Pregnancy*"), the books do contain advice from caregivers.

In this section, we are searching for the "basic truths" (Hart, 1997, p. 122) that emerge about breastfeeding as they are situated in informational texts about the reality of giving birth. We are doing so because "generic patterns stabilize social life" (Hart, 1997, p. 122). The most obvious patterns that emerge in the case of pregnancy and childbirth books is an emphasis on the *heuristic of the natural*. In general, these books demonstrate a preference to all things that occur "naturally," which, of course, includes breastfeeding:

> If you're looking for a practitioner that will put more caring into your ob care, take extra time with you at pre-natal visits, be as attentive to your emotional wellbeing as your physical condition, offer more detailed nutritional advice and comprehensive breast feeding support, be open to more complementary and alternative therapies and more birth options, and be a strong advocate of unmedicated birth, than a certified nurse-midwife may be right for you (though, of course, many doctors fit that profile too). (Murkoff & Mazel, 2016, p. 11)

Syntax and form, as well as message density are of particular note in this excerpt. Who wouldn't want all of the above, especially as advertised? What woman would say "no" to "*more* caring" being put "into" obstetrician and gynecological care? Who would turn down "*extra* care" at prenatal visits, especially considering the vast majority of readers are first time mothers—women for whom the book is created? "*More* detailed nutritional advice?" Yes, please! "*More* comprehensive breastfeeding support" suggests that little will be given at a doctor's office (which may or may not be true). Finally, the passage reveals the belief that natural is better because it is "*more* complimentary." It's hard to imagine a reader denying themselves of any of this, despite the fact that even the book, with a slight tip of the hat, acknowledges that all these things can be found at the presumably "unnatural" doctor's office. The power of this passage relies on the concept of *more*. There is *more* to be gained from the natural than can be offered from the sterility of the medical community.

A similar tactic is used in *Pregnancy:*

> Research shows us that breastfeeding is the very best option for a new baby. Study after study concludes that breastfed babies thrive and outperform on cognitive skill test versus those who were bottle-fed. Nature innately knows how to formulate the right nutrients your child needs. We are aware that in today's world it is challenging to breastfeed your baby until they are naturally weaned. However, we are firmly suggesting you allow three months as the minimum time frame. The

> longer you can breastfeed, the better for your baby. (McAllister, 2017, [Kindle version, location 975])

While *What to Expect* focused on *more*, *Pregnancy* focuses on *better*. And, as we've seen throughout the book, better means natural. The passage begins by framing the message in terms of research (though medical science is often questioned when it doesn't fit the narrative) and *knowing* what is best. If the reader is somehow unaware of that research, they are now duly informed. Cognitive skills are used as a measure of success for children, not overall productivity, health, wellness, and happiness of the adults that they will grow into. A brief nod is given to the difficulties of breastfeeding but is followed directly by a firm suggestion which acts as a rebuttal. The argument's form is clear: Breastfeeding is your "option." It is your only real option, though it is framed in terms of "choice."

This is because *Pregnancy* views breastfeeding as a foregone conclusion, not a choice. Challenges to breastfeeding are viewed as defections, not as credible reasons to bottle feed: "If you experience challenges with breastfeeding, we recommend you contact a lactation consultant" (McAllister, 2017, [Kindle version, location 995]). The author does acknowledge that "in some cases, breastfeeding is not possible," and offers a recipe for an alternative option that includes raw organic egg yolk, cod liver, and pure oil in addition to formula (McAllister, 2017, [Kindle version, location 995]).

Pregnancy says little more about bottle feeding. After the alternative option recipe, the chapter moves on to the use of probiotics while breastfeeding, once again reinforcing the heuristic of the natural as a means to healthy pregnancies and babies. In general, pregnancy and childbirth books speak volumes about breastfeeding but say relatively little about bottle feeding. *What to Expect* provides an interesting example of how a text's unstated priorities can be revealed through an analysis of the presence of absence.

What to Expect adheres to the form of most pregnancy and childbirth books by providing organizational structure through listing (providing a veritable "To-Do List" for expecting readers). These lists provide obvious insight into the book's structural design, but more latently, also reveal the text's message emphasis and density. A "To-Do" list implies that all tasks must be completed in order to achieve success. While many of us often don't finish our To-Do lists, we don't set out to make them because we hope to fail at the things we need to get done. We also experience anxiety if things are not checked off.

What to Expect provides a To-Do List that helps prepare parents for the birth process, while also setting the rules for the birth process. The list suggests that mothers contact "The local La Leche League, especially if breastfeeding support is a priority for you" (Murkoff & Mazel, 2016, p. 15). There is an assumption here that women should contact LLLI anyway—even if support is not a *priority*, a word which in itself is loaded with implications. Noticeably absent—and therefore not given message emphasis—is advice on who to contact or where to find advice on bottles or pumps. The list also doesn't explain that if you are giving birth at a Baby-Friendly Hospital, neither will be automatically provided, but instead must be insisted upon by the mother. That information, the reader will find out later in the passage, is reserved for *What to Expect in the First Year*. While both breastfeeding and bottle feeding are directly related to infant feeding, the former is important enough to include in the "To-Do" list of both books (*What to Expect When You're Expecting* and *What to Expect in the First Year*). The importance of breastfeeding is so great, that an entire page—specially inserted with borders to make it stand out—is dedicated to a section entitled "Breastfeeding while Pregnant" (Murkoff & Mazel, 2016, p. 30). This information functions as something *identifiable* for the reader. All (extra)important pieces of information are constructed this way throughout the book. Readers are led to important concepts through form, syntax, and imagery. By implication, if the information isn't important (it's *what to expect* after all), then there is no need to expect it. Whether by intention or not, the resulting message is that women shouldn't expect to need bottles.

Elimination sequences like these slowly limit reader's options until only one option, posing as "choice," remains. Pregnancy and childbirth books recast cultural feminist narratives and the heuristic of the natural until they become the readily accepted position of the reader. However, for many, breastfeeding is a choice, and perhaps a luxury realistically actualized within class hierarchies. Choice, while articulated as such, is limited through discourse (who wants to be a bad mother) and is specific to the choices privileged women can make.

Economic issues are a reality for most parents, and are addressed in many pregnancy and childbirth books, and justifiably so. Many of us have lost sleep wondering how to make ends meet, particularly when a baby is on the way. In *What to Expect*, economic insecurity is assuaged through breastfeeding. The authors calm the fears of readers who may be asking, "Can we afford a larger family?" (Murkoff & Mazel, 2016, p. 147), by providing a solution: breastfeeding. Breastfeeding is "free." There are no bottles or formula to buy, so parents can rest easy knowing that there is a natural solution to at least one money problem.

While a seemingly obvious argument, it's also fraught with hasty generalizations. For example, breastfeeding mothers have difficulty returning to work without interrupting their milk supply, which means they will either have to wait to return to work, or rely on alternative feeding methods. The average cost of exclusive formula feeding is $70–150.00 per month (BabyCenter.com, 2017). This adds up to $1,800.00 per year, at the most. While a significant cost, particularly for people who are struggling financially, breastfeeding is unlikely to be the financial save-all it's being touted as. It also won't cover the loss of a mother's paycheck. Health care coverage in the United States can also affect infant feeding. Women without it may not have access to lactation consultants should they have trouble with breastfeeding—which many do. In this sense, learning to breastfeed may be considered yet another class-based issue. If a woman doesn't qualify for WIC, but also doesn't have insurance at their jobs (a benefit they also would lose if they chose not to return to work in order to stay home to exclusively breastfeed), they also will encounter difficulties in procuring a lactation consultant. In short, women who fall in the economic limbo between poor and middle class have limited choices when it comes to infant feeding.

Pregnancy and childbirth books are perhaps the best concrete examples of discursive formations we've presented in this book. They are physical examples of rule sets for mothering. The rules become clear, because these books are planning out motherhood for us. They are showing us how to do it. In this sense, once again, absence becomes very important. Some of the common characteristics in our analysis of the genre reveal that most pregnancy and childbirth books contain the following: 1) Suggestions for birth plans include breastfeeding help, but not bottle feeding suggestions; 2) When choosing a pediatrician, mothers should ask about breastfeeding support (see page 343 of *What to Expect,* for example); and 3) assumptions that mothers will breastfeed if possible from the start, and hopefully continue past three months.

The latter of these characteristics is the tough sell. As we've demonstrated, many mothers give breastfeeding a try, but few continue beyond the first three months. *What to Expect*'s "Chapter 16: Post-partum: The First Week" sets out to correct this. This chapter begins a 10-page discussion of breastfeeding. Prominent topics include breastfeeding as a "fat flattener," breast milk that "keeps allergies on hold" and works as a "brain booster," and appeals to the natural with assurances that "it's safe," and "made for suckers" (Murkoff & Mazel, 2016, p. 566). Breast milk is also a "convenience," and once again, "money in the bank." The entire section on breastfeeding emphasizes the "rightness" of breastfeeding through its naturalness. Moreover, the section includes the composition of breast milk, but ignores what happens if the mother isn't getting enough nutrients, only offering the mother a vague suggestion to eat right and be nutritious for her baby. Additionally, this section of the book makes formula seem extremely inconvenient. It articulates that with breastfeeding mothers have "no formula to run out of, shop for, or lug around, no bottles to clean or refill, no powders to mix, no meals to warm" (Murkoff & Mazel, 2016, p. 368). However, absent from this idyllic portrayal of breastfeeding is the cost of a nursing bra, a breast pump, and navigating where to use it and/or feed a baby from the breast. Nor is the pain of mastitis discussed, the visits to lactation consultants (and the time a woman has to budget to do go), or the bags and freezer storage needed to keep expressed milk cold at work. There are potential dangers of breast milk, particularly when not expressed properly or when women are undernourished. None of these things are mentioned as potential issues with breastfeeding. Doing it right is just assumed.

What to Expect includes a special in-lay in its breastfeeding section labeled "When Father knows Breast." The in-lay explains to first time dads that the breast isn't just sexual. It's functional. The in-lay goes on to explain the benefits of breast milk: "Without a doubt, the decision to choose breast over bottle can make a dramatic difference in your baby's life—and your partners" (Murkoff & Mazel, 2016, p. 739). There is no explanation of what the authors mean by "dramatic." Finally, fathers learn that mothers are far more likely to try breastfeeding if their partners want them to or at least support them. The insert tells husbands to be advocates. To encourage their partner, even if she is tired . . .

Or, we could be left to our own devices, as grown, functional adults. But that argument is for another chapter! The difficulties that these mothers will endure while breastfeeding is left out of this vital information for first-time fathers. Message pacing makes the process of breastfeeding seem idyllic—if I breastfeed, everything will be calm, natural, and easy. But it won't be. Pregnancy and childbirth books are woefully lean on topics like chapped nipples, babies that won't latch, inability to feed due to illness, circumstance, and other difficulties. All of these situations are real and revert back to the heuristic of the natural discussed earlier. Much like Schlafly's portrayal of the natural frustrations of "the journey" of motherhood (see chapter 2), the absence and/or downplaying of the difficulties of breastfeeding render them as natural realities that good mothers accept and endure. In contrast, the difficulties associated with bottle feeding are constructed as unnecessary "interruptions," a word used throughout *What to Expect* and articulated in similar ways in *Pregnancy,* when discussing the medical and scientific processes of modern delivery.

The idyllic picture portrayed through the heuristic of the natural breaks down when the realities of motherhood present themselves: "And if you and your baby aren't in the same place at the same time—you're away at work, in school, at dinner, or even away for the weekend—a stash of expressed milk can be served up in bottles" (Murkoff & Mazel, 2016, p. 568). So . . . bottles *will* be required (not included on the list of things to bring to the hospital) . . . and will have to be cleaned and sanitized. Also, expressed milk assumes you have the supply to use milk your baby doesn't need at the time of feeding. For Jenni, each ounce of milk she made was necessary at the time of feeding. And she couldn't make enough to feed her sons as they grew. Her experience is not uncommon, but not addressed in pregnancy and childbirth books.

What to Expect offers a more comprehensive look at breastfeeding. While not explicitly a pregnancy and childbirth book, it does begin by explaining the first moments of life. An insert on "Feeding Time" starts out like this: "Remember how you timed your contractions—counting from the beginning of one to the beginning of the next? Good—because you'll be timing breastfeeding sessions the same way" (p. 480). Pages are dedicated to showing the how to's, the holds, when to wake a baby up, how to encourage the baby to feed, what to do for babies who have problems feeding, etc. There is no such instruction for bottle feeding.

What to Expect in the First Year reads much the same as *What to Expect When You're Expecting*: tips for breastfeeding, myth busters, why breast milk is the "best" and "easiest" food for your baby, etc. There is a half-page insert that provides small solitude to the mother who can't or chooses not, to breastfeed. Entitled "When you Can't or Shouldn't Breastfeed" (not "When you decide not to Breastfeed") the insert "debunks" the valid reasons for not breastfeeding (i.e., lets women know how they can breastfeed, even if they've been told they shouldn't). Most of the tips require more work from the mother. At the end of the insert, the authors say: "But if you can't or shouldn't breastfeed (or don't want to), not to worry, not to feel guilty, not to stress, not to regret. The right formula can nourish your baby well—as will the love you offer with that bottle" (Murkoff & Mazel, 2014, p. 4). The small insert, that really serves to let women who've been told not to breastfeed how they should and can, offers this last bit of support for mothers in a manner which is too little, and based on the sheer lack of attention to these mothers, demeaning. Mothers deserve all the options available to them, not just those that some people prefer.

In each book, with the exception of *Pregnancy* which all but ignores bottle feeding, the section on formula feeding (if included) is provided *after* the section on breastfeeding. The section is always smaller, but similarly constructed (i.e., benefits, things to think about, and things to expect/prepare for). Bottle feeding's placement after breastfeeding reveals its place of preference. Is bottle feeding okay? Sure (now that it might be a reality for the reader). But it's not ideal. Not because formula can't properly nourish a child, but because it's not "natural." In *What to Expect in the First Year*, the bottle feeding section is followed by "Your Feelings:" "Maybe you're convinced by the fact [that breastfeeding is best], but nagging doubts are still keeping you on the breastfeeding fence. Here's how to work through a few common negative feelings about breastfeeding" (Murkoff & Mazel, 2014, p. 9). The wording, and placement of the text (sandwiching bottle feeding in-between breastfeeding discourses) serves as a reinforcement of breastfeeding. The section also relegates breastfeeding and bottle feeding to feelings. Problematically, discourses of motherhood reinforce selflessness and sacrifice. The moment we give birth, and for most of us, the moment we realize we are pregnant, our feelings are no longer ours. They don't matter anymore. We are mothers. Our feelings, unless they are in direct relation to our children, are simply things that get in the way of our duty. These books tell us "not to worry.

We will help you!" Help, however, comes in the form of reinforcement and backhanded shaming. Rather than simply leaving the mother be, trusting her to her own feelings and desires and reiterating that those feelings and desire are okay, the book says, "just try it." Literally: "Before you write off breastfeeding entirely, here's a suggestion: Try it. You may like it. You might even love it" (Murkoff & Mazel, 2014, p. 9). If you don't love it, you tried and you gave baby all those amazing benefits. Every feed counts" (Murkoff & Mazel, 2014, p. 9). Really? Every feed? How much does it count? Explain. Because until this point in the reading, all the information has suggested otherwise. Readers have been explicitly told to exclusively breastfeed for the first year, or their babies will suffer.

In the end, though, these books do give a nod to mothers who don't breastfeed. In doing so, they get to the heart of what we are trying to say with this book:

> But if you choose not to breastfeed, or you can't breastfeed, or you can or choose to breastfeed only for the briefest of times, there's no need for second guessing, regret, or guilt. Almost nothing you do for your baby is right if it doesn't end up feeling right for you—and that includes breastfeeding. A bottle offered lovingly is better for your little one than a breast offered with reservations, or a side of stress. (Murkoff & Mazel, 2014, p. 10)

We wholeheartedly agree. But perhaps the discussion should start off with this, not end with it.

The Mayo Clinic Guide to a Healthy Pregnancy is a bit more balanced in how it presents infant feeding information. The section on infant feeding begins with a thoughtful progression of possibilities:

> Some women know right from the start what they'll do—breast-feed or bottle-feed—while others struggle. Most child health organization advocate breast-feeding, and "breast is best" is a commonly used phrase. There's no doubt, breast-feeding is a wonderful way to nourish a newborn—breast milk provides numerous benefits. Mayo Clinic experts agree.
>
> However, care providers also realize that not all women are the same, and people's life situations are different. Depending on your circumstances, certain factors may lead you to choose infant formula instead of breast milk. Or you may opt for a combination of both breast milk and formula.
>
> Some women who choose the bottle instead of the breast are bothered by their decision. They worry they're not being a good mother or putting the needs of their child first. If you're among this group, don't shower yourself in guilt. Such negative thinking isn't good for you—or for your baby.
>
> Feeding, regardless of how it's delivered—breast milk or formula, breast or bottle—promotes intimacy.

> Know that both options will provide your child the nutrition he or she needs to grow and thrive. (Wick, 2018, [Kindle version, location 69])

This discussion veers from other pregnancy and childbirth books. Its balance offers a more comprehensive look at breastfeeding possibilities than the other books we've analyzed in this section. Mayo's *Guide* tells women to talk with care providers to determine what is best for their situation. The *Guide* also suggests being prepared for both feeding methods at the time of birth and to think through other situational factors like work and relationships when considering infant care options. In all, Mayo's *Guide* is a more detailed discussion—and a more precise/research-based discussion—of infant feeding. Still, the information on breastfeeding is vastly more detailed in form and content than bottle feeding. Twenty-eight pages are dedicated to breastfeeding and involve intimate discussions of particular infant holds, nipple pain, breast discomfort, and the like. In contrast, only fifteen pages are dedicated to bottle feeding. Nonetheless, unlike the other books in this section, the Mayo *Guide* is careful to point out the pros and cons of each method and in sum, provides a more balanced and thorough discussion of infant feeding. This is a trend we hope to expand with this book because while Mayo's *Guide*, is a popular choice for mothers, it is far outsold by *What to Expect*. We are pleased that there is a book that balances the pros and cons of breastfeeding and formula feeding, yet it is not the primary mothering guide reaching new and expecting mothers/people (Pederson & Effron, 2012).

We are not suggesting that the ideal is bad. As we state throughout the book, breastfeeding discourses exist within a context of neoliberal ideology, and as such, tend to disarticulate women's experiences from their lived realities (and the multiple realities of family and feeding practices). Breastfeeding is constructed as perfect and awesome, and amazing, and even easy. *It is natural*. But as McRobbie (2009) explains, there is a "punitive response to being shown to those who live outside the economic unit of the two parent family" (p. 6). Breastfeeding is depicted as a reality that exists between a man, a woman, and their child. So when it all comes to a head, and it's (the breast, the mother, the family, etc.) not any or all of these things, what do women do? We rush, we worry, and we cry—we recognize we are not part of the conversation taking place (gay fathers, for example). Talking about alternatives to breastfeeding doesn't result in unhealthy or deceased babies. It's a way to insure mothers and parents understand they will be fine—and so will their babies—if things don't go as easily as advertised.

NOTE

1. We use the term "author-ities" as it relates to Foust's (2008) use of the term in her article Aesthetics as Weapons in the "War of Ideas:" Exploring the Digital and Typographic in American Conservative Web Sites. *Southern Communication Journal, 73,* 2, 122–42.

FIVE

Disciplining the Marginalized Maternal Body

Discourses of Race, Class, and Privilege

The breast-is-best movement in the United States has historically been constructed as a breast-is-best-if-you're-a-white-middle-class-educated-professional woman. That is the privileged position that the two of us authors occupy. With that said, we also recognize that absent from much of the pro-breastfeeding discourse are matters related to race/ethnicity, SES, sexual orientation, and occupation. These intersecting identities are the focus of this chapter. We will begin our chapter with a discussion of the whiteness embedded in current breastfeeding practices and discourses and, by extension, in the construct of hegemonic mothering. Thereafter, we will unpack further the racist, heterosexist, and classist nature of the *statistics discourse* about who is and who is not breastfeeding and how the *barriers to breastfeeding* discourse contain these biases. Our intent is to expose a matrix of domination (Collins, 1990) wherein social position impacts both the constraints and privileges of breastfeeding.

First, however, we wish to acknowledge more deeply our own positionality and how that impacts our review of this discourse. As stated, we are white, heterosexual, middle-class, educated women. It is through this privileged cisgendered lens that we examine matters related to the breastfeeding experiences of women who have backgrounds different from our own. We do not intend to speak for these women; instead, we recognize that we are seeking to reveal the discourse of disparities as through our own white, feminist eyes. Where possible, we include voices of women of color themselves, elevating their own and quieting our own white authorial tone. In so doing, we wish to lay bare our own privileges as cisgendered, middle-class white women and white mothers, in particular. We know that, as women of these positionalities, we too have been a part of a system of domination and oppression (Collins, 1990; hooks, 2015) that has marginalized and silenced mothers of color and from working class backgrounds. It is precisely this lived experience that motivates our desire to speak with and not for mothers of all backgrounds and creeds. bell hooks (2015) reminds us that

> Moving from silence into speech is for the oppressed, the colonized, the exploited, and those who stand struggle side by side a gesture of defiance that heals, that makes new life and new growth possible. It is that act of speech, of "talking back," that is no mere gesture of empty words, that is the expression of our movement from object to subject—the liberated voice. (p. 9)

We begin this multi-vocal, liberating journey of talking back with an interrogation of the whiteness embedded in the pro-breastfeeding ideology and entangled in hegemonic mothering. This section is followed by an analysis of two discursive formations (Foucault, 2010a) that expose racial and class biases in the science of breastfeeding. We argue that similar to hegemonic femininity (Favre, 2015), hegemonic motherhood is couched in the privileged discourses of white, upper-middle class, heteronormative feminine experience, "functioning to situate white middle-class women as guardians of national civility" (Favre, 2015, p. 629). Moreover, we intend to provide insight into how the ability for mobility, both physically and within class systems, provide wealthy white women more "choices" in enacting motherhood, and as such, "create financial qualifications for motherhood" (Favre, 2015, p. 634).

THE PRESENCE OF ABSENCE: WHITENESS IN THE PRO-BREASTFEEDING MOVEMENT

Breasts may be best for babies, but the realities of difficult racial histories in the United States render monolithic initiatives rather ineffective, and often, insulting. As Baer (2016) explains, neo-liberal discourses "create a situation of permanent insecurity that disproportionately affects minority groups" (p. 21). For women of color, breastfeeding discourses have always reflected white realities, and, as a result, these women often experience difficulties in "measuring up" to the white rules that define good and bad mothering. Breastfeeding policies and initiatives like those analyzed in chapter 3 often do not mark the mother's or baby's race or SES unless the mother/baby is of color and from a working-class background. Hence, the "mother" is assumed to be white and middle-to-upper class. Through the absence of labeling, the one who is present is the white mother. All others are judged as different and, many times, as underperforming their maternal duties. Consequently, they become the subjects of the medi-institutionalized gaze which surveils them most frequently and polices them most harshly (Foucault, 1994; 1995). Granted, as the pro-breastfeeding movement has become medicalized and institutionalized, all new mothers must function within a panoptical reality, observed, judged, and disciplined by those in charge (Foucault, 1994; 1995) and society at large. For *disciplinary power*, according to Foucault,

> is exercised through its invisibility; at the same time it imposes on those whom it subjects a principle of compulsory visibility. In discipline, it is the subjects who have to be seen. Their visibility assures the hold of the power that is exercised over them. It is the fact of constantly being seen, of being able always to be seen, that maintains the disciplined individual in his [sic] subjection. (p. 187)

Yet, even within the panoptican (Foucault, 1995) exists a hierarchy, and in ours, mothers of color and lower SES find themselves most vulnerable to scrutiny and most susceptible to the gaze. The absence of race and class markings allows the white mother to be both the norm by which all others are judged while simultaneously escaping some of the additional scrutiny that accompanies her subject position as a body to be monitored and disciplined should her race be marked.

Part of white women's privileged mother subjectivity is the power to define motherhood—even in instances when they mother children of color. For example, privileged mothers like Angelina Jolie who adopt international children from underprivileged parts of the world are rearticulating what it means to be a mother. These "global mothers," who are saving and rescuing disadvantaged children are, according to Shome (2011), recentering "white Western (and especially North Atlantic) heterosexual kinship logics" (p. 389). So, even in instances involving children of color, the white, adoptive global mother becomes the ideal by which all moms are judged, thereby erasing the possibility that others may occupy this highly valued subject position.

While white women are able to transcend national boundaries and coopt the meaning of mother, women of color are typically not afforded such luxuries. This is certainly true within our own country and most clearly with black mothers. While well intentioned, breastfeeding narratives often:

> contribute to contemporary mothering rhetorics that reinforce hierarchical distinctions among and between mothers. Public discourses about Black women breastfeeding draw upon complex histories of race/ racism, sexism, and U.S. governmentality and work as cultural forces that elicit advice, support, insult, and disdain. The practice of breastfeeding and its public negotiation, even when supportive, is about surveilling and disciplining women's bodies (Bartlett, 2003) and contributes to the ways that Black motherhood has historically come to be seen as suspect. (Morrissey & Kimball, 2017, pp. 49–50)

Breastfeeding discourses "*about* Black motherhood that have circulated throughout the U.S. cultural imaginary have constructed Black women as bad mothers who, among other failings, do not breastfeed their children as they are supposed to" (Morrissey & Kimball, 2017, p. 50, emphasis added). Morrissey and Kimball (2017) assert that breastfeeding narratives have historically served in "redirecting Black mothers' breast milk *away from* Black infants and *toward* some wealthy White mothers" (p. 49).

Breastfeeding initiatives that we have reviewed in this book have been set to meet the realities of a specific type of mother. Upon examination, that mother, who while never mentioned within the discourses surrounding *why* breastfeeding should take place, looks very white. The assumption of white heteronormativity embedded within the medical-institutionalized discourse reviewed in chapter 3, for example, places women of color in a double-bind that keeps them outside of breastfeeding initiatives and thus constructions of good motherhood.

Importantly, mothers of color have begun to talk back (hooks, 2015) to these raced presuppositions about breastfeeding, making themselves more visible in the public sphere. While we will explore more of these discourses of resistance in chapter 7, we do want to provide a glimpse into their oppositional, resistance discourse. These types of movements and projects are ways the women of color are pushing back against the whiteness contained within hegemonic mothering. For instance, Kimberly Seals Allers' Mocha Manual,[1] The Black Mothers' Breastfeeding Association,[2] Salud America,[3] and Mommys Wall for Indian mothers[4] are just some of the sites that women of color have created and turn to for breastfeeding guidance. A strong theme among the discourse on these sites is the need for cultural awareness—the need for individual women within these cultures to be the ones talking to other moms because the white medi-insitutionalized policy discourse does not speak for them. As such, many women of color have found alternative spaces where they can talk about infant feeding in a culturally specific way. And, perhaps, these spaces are ways in which women of color can resist the pressure to assimilate into the world of white, medi-institutionalized, racist supremacy (hooks, 2015).

One such action began on August 25, 2013, when black breastfeeding advocates worked together to create the first Black Breastfeeding Week (BBW). The goal of this campaign was (and is) to raise awareness within the black community about breastfeeding and parenting, in general. From our vantage point, it was also a form of resistance and counter hegemonic discourse.

BBW co-founder Anayah Sangodele-Ayoka (Swanson, 2013), stated in an interview, "When we deal with a larger culture that positions breastfeeding as something white women do—or at least something specifically not black [that is a challenge]. The larger narrative is about white women, so even physicians don't address it." She went on to add, "It's not about physiology; it's about social context." Part of that historical social context for African American women's feelings toward breastfeeding is, in part, because "black women have always worked outside of the home, quite often as domestic help for white families—caring for white children—and that formula was supposed to make it easier for them to be separated from their own babies."

It is our hope that, as these discourses of resistance become louder, as we as a society begin to respect the varied ways that motherhood is enacted, and as the white ideal embedded in hegemonic mothering is noticed and challenged, true change can occur. We are inspired by bell hooks (2015) who stated,

> When we dare to speak in a liberatory voice, we threaten even those who may initially claim to want our words. In the act of overcoming our fear of speech, of being seen as threatening, in the process of learning to speak as subjects, we participate in the global struggle to end domination. (p. 18)

Sadly, as we discuss in our next section, we are not there yet. Instead, as the politics of our country shifted in its pro-female ideology and governments and health care facilities began to institutionalize breastfeeding, the woman's body has become more and more an object of subjection (Rabinow, 1984, p. 7). One of Foucault's mode of objectification that is particularly applicable here is the process by which a subject is objectified via "dividing practices"—known as "modes of manipulation that combine the mediation of science (or pseudo-science) and the practice of exclusion" (Rabinow, 1984, p. 8). Not only has the woman's breast been separated from her body, but the institutional discourse also has corresponded to the increase scientific examination of the differences *between* women. This "scientific classification" (Foucault's second form of objectification, Rabinow, 1984) of mothers is especially relevant when it comes to comparing them across racial and class lines.

THE RACIALIZED AND CLASSIST DISCOURSE OF BREASTFEEDING RESEARCH: STATISTICS

It has been said many times that statistics don't lie, which can be true. But, they can also be manipulated to represent the researcher's point of view. Science, after all, is not neutral but instead contains ideological perspectives that vary in their opaqueness. It may seem impossible for there to be a connection between biology (lactation) and ideology (breast is best) because science is thought to be value free. However, science as an institution is not a neutral system of meaning. Rather, it is embedded with particular ideologies, all struggling for legitimacy. Ideology, or a way of looking at the world, can lead to domination by the belief that the empirical-medical-scientific gaze is superior to the subjective. According to Foucault (1994), "medical rationality plunges into the marvelous density of perception, offering the grain of things as the first face of truth" (p. xiii). Science is one such ideological system which, when left unchecked, forms the structures of Knowledge. The observing eye of the science, or the empirical gaze, "becomes the depositary and source of clarity" (Foucault, 1994, p. xiii).

There is a large amount of science examining breastfeeding. We assert that the language of this science forms a certain type of discursive formation that privileges white mothers' subjectivity as the norm by which all other mothers are compared, sometimes conceals differences between white women and mothers of color while other times emphasizing them. As such, the ideology embedded in the statistics discourse is one more facet of hegemonic mothering. Institutionalized medical discourse, in particular, turns the gaze to the body (Foucault, 1994), and in our case, to the woman's body—a body to be surveilled, disciplined, and punished.

Key statistics discourses can be found in several of the (quasi) government documents reviewed in chapter 3. Specifically, they often contain summaries of breastfeeding research, including statistics about who and who is not breastfeeding. Much of the language surrounding the statistics discourse is about the *goals for breastfeeding*—pitting mothers against one another and determining *for* them what their goals should be.

Classifying Mothers

Numerous government agencies, such as the CDC and Health and Human Services, track breastfeeding rates among women. In addition, demographic variables such as marital status, income, education, race, age, and poverty/level are most often measured. For example, the U.S. Department of Health and Human Services' Healthy People 2010 initiative set national goals for breastfeeding. These goals included 75 percent of all women having "ever" breastfed, 50 percent "at six months," and 25 percent "at 12 months." In reviewing the findings, the discourse often highlights what goals were met and which ones were not—by whom and not by whom. For instance, there is talk about the only objective that was met was the *average* initiation rate of 75 percent across *all* mothers. Discussion continues by noting that African American women were the one specific racial group that did not meet this goal, with approximately 60 percent (compared to the average of 75 percent) reported having initiated breastfeeding while in the hospital.

In the governmental documents, after presenting the classification statistics about who and who is not breastfeeding, the discourse typically switches to the "disparities" in breastfeeding practices *between* white and women of color, African American women most commonly. For example, in the Call to Action (The Surgeon General's, 2011), it is noted that even when controlling for family income and educational level, the rates of breastfeeding black infants are approximately 50 percent lower than for white babies at birth, 6 months, and 12 months. Many scholars have noted similar trends. Jones, Power, Queenan, and Schulkin (2015), for instance, assert that African American women have historically had the lowest rates of breastfeeding initiation and continuation and are 2.5 times less likely to breastfeed than white women.

What often goes unexamined in this statistics discourse is that, in contrast to black and white mothers, Asian and Hispanic women have the highest rates (Jones et al., 2015)! Specifically, Asian and Hispanic mothers' breastfeeding initiation rates were 86.4 percent and 80.6 percent, respectively. These rates were higher than the 2010 Healthy People Goals. What is even more interesting is that Asian women were the only ones to *exceed* the 2010 goals for continuing to breastfeed at 6 (58.6 percent) and 12 (34.8 percent) months. If we round up, Hispanic mothers also met the goal of 25 percent breastfeeding at 12 months.

Also, the CDC's Healthy People 2020 objectives are approximately 82 percent for breastfeeding initiation, 61 percent for continued breastfeeding at 6 months, and 34 percent at 12 months. Once again Asian women are the only racial/ethnic group meeting the initiation goal of 81.9 percent with Hispanic women very close to meeting this number. No group is meeting the 2020 goals for continuing to breastfeed at 6 and 12 months.

Nowhere in the general breastfeeding discourse is it seriously acknowledged that Asian and Hispanic mothers breastfeed more than other women. Nor is there a legitimate attempt to understand how and why these women, in particular, have such high breastfeeding rates. Their subject positions of women of color gets erased in the assumed white norm. Moreover, the myopic focus on white mothers compared to black mothers exacerbates the pained historical relationship between the two groups of women and creates an even larger psychic wound as black mothers continue to be defined by white women.

The classifactory gaze (Foucault, 1995) embedded in the statistics discourse functions as a dividing practice which both objectifies and differentiates the subjects (the mothers) (Foucault, 1995). On one hand, the mothers' bodies are subordinated to the social institutions of science and medicine; "the constituted subject can be seen as a victim caught in the process of objectification and constraint" (Rabinow, 1984, p. 11). Yet, by an absence of labeling, white mothers remain the group by which all other mothers are measured—even when some women of color "outperform" them. Black women are compared to white women; Asian and Hispanic mothers are reduced to numbers and thereby erased of human subjectivity. Even though Hispanic and Asian mothers are breastfeeding at higher rates than white mothers, they never become the reference group—the liberated body.

Erasing Mothers

While much of the governmental statistics discourse focuses attention on the differences between mothers, other reports erase the mothers and emphasize the actions of the *babies*. For example, in a recent CDC report, entitled *Racial and Geographic Differences in Breastfeeding—United States, 2011–2015* (Anstey, Chen, Elam-Evans, & Perrine, 2017), the results from a National Immunization Survey were analyzed. The *infants* who had the highest rates of initiated breastfeeding, included those who were Hispanic (81.9 percent) or white, non-Hispanic (81.5 percent) with a college educated mother who was at least 30 years of age or older and did not qualify for WIC because the family income was at least 600 percent or more above the poverty level. Conversely, the characteristics of the *infants* with the lowest rates of initiated breastfeeding were those who were black, non-Hispanic (64.3 percent) and whose mother was less than 20 years of age, had less than a high school diploma or GED, qualified for WIC, and lived below the poverty level.

There are several points to make regarding the framing of these statistics. First, it is important for us to make clear that, on one hand, we appreciate the fact that so many agencies are examining breastfeeding patterns. But, beyond knowing that, we really don't understand much more about the how and why behind these numbers nor about the maternal body as an agentic being. Instead the result of this type of discursive formation is that mothers are reduced to a set of variables and, sometimes, in the case of the disparities between race study, they are erased altogether. The focus once again turns to the child and the act of breastfeeding. In addition, when mother-centric factors, such as age, education, or race, are examined, those variables dominate the narrative. Black mothers don't breastfeed. Uneducated mothers don't breastfeed. Poor women don't. Conversely, White and Hispanic mothers do as do women with higher educations and incomes. This discourse focused on the differences between mothers, like many of the mommy wars, pits women against each other. It also keeps the focus on the problem with women and creates a hierarchy of good and bad mothering based upon a set of demographic variables.

Moreover, the classifactory gaze (Foucault, 1994), which focuses on breastfeeding rates, perpetuates a discourse that monitors which mothers are complying with the pro-breastfeeding ideology and which ones are not. Their visibility becomes the means for disciplining (Foucault, 1995) them into compliance and punishing those who do not. This brand of disciplinary power, of being seen and monitored, maintains the disciplined mother in her subjection (Foucault, 1995). All mothers, as studied and classified bodies, are subjected to this discipline, but it is the women of color and those from working class backgrounds who are declared the non-conformists and punished for being bad, deviant, and deficient. As we will demonstrate in the coming pages, since most pro-breastfeeding goals remain unmet, the classifactory gaze quickly changes to the barriers *to* breastfeeding.

THE RACIALIZED AND CLASSIST DISCOURSE OF BREASTFEEDING RESEARCH BARRIERS

Along with the pro-breastfeeding and research discourses found in the quasi-governmental and governmental agencies' documents discussed earlier in this chapter and in depth in chapter 3, these same organizations also present various "barriers to breastfeeding." An analysis of the barriers discourse reveals more layers embedded within hegemonic mothering—in this case, we are reminded that it is women of color and those from working class backgrounds who are the bad mothers because they cannot overcome the challenges to breastfeeding. To draw once again from McRobbie (2009), there is an assumption of equality in most governmental discourses (i.e., discourses assume gender equality on their face) but despite strident feminist activism, particularly from the 1960s and 1970s, the system didn't change enough to operationalize full scale equality (e.g., we can't breastfeed past 12 weeks because we have to go back to work). Women, and particularly women of color and women from lower socio-economic backgrounds, were allowed to play the game of work, but the game didn't change to let any of us play fairly. Dual gendered discourses gave us purchasing power—not equality.

Marking

The hierarchical ordering of mothers is most evidenced by how the non-dominant culture is often linguistically marked (black mother) while the dominant white culture is not (mother). Racial and ethnic differences are often highlighted when discussing impediments to breastfeeding. By marking women of color and/or with lower income backgrounds in this way, they are framed as the ones who have "the problems." The implication then is that it is primarily black mothers and those who are working class who are violating the expectations of what it means to be a good mother in our society. It needs to be reiterated that Asian mothers have the highest breastfeeding rates, but that fact is never linguistically noted. Nor are white women marked when discussing the barriers to breastfeeding. As a result, because of their privileged racial position and the absence of identifying race, white mothers are assumed to be the ones with the highest breastfeeding rates and the least amount of problems trying to do so—in other words, the best mothers.

Here is one case in point. In The Call (The Surgeon General's, 2011) discussed previously in chapter 3, the following are noted as *Barriers to*

Breastfeeding in the United States: lack of knowledge, social norms, poor family and social support, embarrassment, lactation problems, employment and child care, and barriers related to health services. For starters, even the barrier labels using words such as *lack, poor, embarrassment,* and *problems* immediately frame mothers as inadequate, uneducated, and weak and their families as nonsupportive. The discussion becomes even more biased when examining the language within each barrier.

Throughout the larger discussion of barriers, the words *mother* and *women* are used frequently. However, only when discussing specific mothers' barriers are the words *low-income, immigrant, low-income Hispanic, African American families* used. For instance, in the section entitled Lack of Knowledge, the following statement is made:

> Unfortunately, education about breastfeeding is not always readily available to mothers nor easily understood by them. Many women rely on books, leaflets, and other written materials as their only source of information on breastfeeding, but using these sources to gain knowledge about breastfeeding can be ineffective, especially for *low-income women, (emphasis added)* who may have more success relying on role models. (The Surgeon General's, 2011, p. 11)

In other words, many mothers suffer from a lack of knowledge about breastfeeding because of the source from which they draw their information. But, low-income women, in particular, seem to have even more trouble reading this information and learning from it. Instead they must rely on a role model to *tell* them the information because they are unable to read it for themselves. This statement makes a very dangerous connection between income and literacy. It is a big leap to infer that a mother who is in the lower income levels of our society is also illiterate and dependent upon oral instruction. Yes, income and literacy may be correlated but there are many other reasons why low-income mothers may not breastfeed—ones that may have more to do with societal structural issues (e.g., employer demand, the lack of a mother-friendly work environment, inadequate health care, low health care efficacy) than their own capacity to consume information.

Another example of marking non-white mothers is included in the Social Norms section of The Call (The Surgeon General's, 2011):

> Certain cultural beliefs and practices also contribute to what women consider to be normal feeding practices, although some of these practices are not recommended today. The mistaken belief that, for babies, "big is healthy," can lead to both formula feeding and inappropriate early introduction of solid foods. *The false idea that larger babies are healthier is common among many racial and ethnic groups (emphasis added),* and mothers who are a part of social networks that hold this belief may be encouraged to supplement breastfeeding with formula if the infant is perceived as thin. (p. 11)

Writing it in this way turns the gaze toward women of color and frames the matter as a problem within non-white racial and non-European ethnic groups. In other words, non-white, non-European mothers are the ones whose cultural beliefs and practices are deficient to the white, European maternal norm.

Fathers of color are marked in similar ways. For instance, in the Poor Family and Social Support barrier The Call it is noted that

> in many families, fathers play a role in the decision of whether to breastfeed. . . . Studies of *African American families (emphasis added)* in which education on breastfeeding was directed at the father found a 20 percent increase in breastfeeding rates, indicating that paternal influences on maternal feeding practices are critically important in early decision making about breastfeeding. (The Surgeon General's, 2011, p. 12)

Don't get us wrong; we're glad that researchers found ways in which fathers can become a more integral part of a mother's decision to formula or breastfeed. Yet, we also find problematic that during a discussion of fathers' role in breastfeeding that African American families are the ones showcased. This frame perpetuates the stereotype of the absent African American dad, showing how much better his family would be if he were there. Interestingly, race is not mentioned in the next paragraph when discussing the findings from two randomized trials examining fathers' *positive* influence on their partners' initiation and duration of breastfeeding. The take away message from this section is that non-racialized fathers (aka white) can have positive influences on breastfeeding, while it takes proper education for African American fathers, more specifically, to have such an impact.

We would be remiss if we did not highlight the heteronormativity embedded in the described expectations for the parental roles. Nowhere in the discussion of barriers are issues that may be unique to gay, lesbian, or trans parents. Nor is the practice of breastfeeding adequately "problematized as gendered or related to heteronormative institutions" (Rippey & Falconi, 2017, p. 16). Like straight parents, non-heterosexual parents all struggle with matters related to breast or bottle feeding. However, there are unique, complex intersections between their gender, sexual orientation, and the biological act of breastfeeding. For example, in a study of transmasculine individuals' (born female and later developed a male gender identity) experiences with lactation, chestfeeding, and gender identity, MacDonald and colleagues (2016), describe how a few participants considered the type and timing of chest masculinization surgery when contemplating pregnancy. Several individuals stated that "the level of gender dysphoria during pregnancy would have been unbearable if they had female-appearing mammary tissue" (p. 5). These perspectives are typically left out of heteronormative parenting classes, books, and even governmental policies. As a result, many of these parents are erased from this conversation and thereby erased from parenting/mothering.

Who's Responsible—Shifting the Blame to Mothers

Speaking of erased, the reader is now familiar with our argument about pro-breastfeeding discourse—that mothers are erased; their agency is stripped, breasts exist outside of women's bodies; and babies are to be treated like the Christ Child! Importantly, however, that perspective is most evident within the discourse *advocating* breastfeeding or the statistics discourse examining breastfeeding rates. In contrast, when discussing the *barriers* to breastfeeding, the conversational tone changes: the mother becomes the agent at fault for not having enough knowledge, not following the proper social norms, and not resisting feelings of embarrassment. This is especially true for women of color, lower education, and/or working class. In addition to this pattern being found in the governmental research documents, it can also be found in academic, peer reviewed research. For instance, in 2015, Jones, Power, Queenan, and Schulkin conducted a systematic review of the research examining the racial and ethnic disparities in breastfeeding rates as well as the barriers reported. They created a list of 16 barriers relevant for this group of women. The barriers and the corresponding labels that the researchers created frame the issue in the same biased way as the government documents. For instance, the beginning of this list of barriers (*Preference to bottle feed, Pain, Discomfort, Inconvenience, and Lack of time)* imply that the mothers are "not trying hard enough." Still others (*Lack of parental knowledge regarding breastfeeding practices, Lack of maternal access to information the promotes and supports breastfeeding, Sexual perceptions, Lifestyle choices, including smoking, alcohol use, and the desire of younger women who want to be independent and free to leave their infant in the care of others, Difficulty with the baby latching onto the breast, and Inadequate milk production)* suggest that there's something wrong with the mother. Additional ones, such as the *Lack of social and cultural acceptance, Lack of support from family, peers, work, and the health care community, and Acculturation,* suggest that the mother's cultural background and/or family are inferior. There is only one socio-structural barrier noted, *Employment,* that acknowledges the structural inequities that impact a woman's ability to breastfeed. Otherwise, all other barriers place the reason for the inadequacy on the mothers or their families. The scientific gaze focuses on them, making them most visible and, hence, subject to disciplining.

For the disciplinary power to function among these women, they must be subjected to more monitoring. One such way this is happening is the numerous initiatives (and governmental dollars) to increase black women's breastfeeding rates as well as mothers living at or below the poverty line. For instance, breastfeeding has become a high priority within the WIC program. According to the U.S. Department of Agriculture's Food and Nutrition Service (United States, 2018),

> WIC mothers are strongly encouraged to breastfeed their infants unless there is a medical reason not to. All WIC staff are trained to promote breastfeeding and provide the necessary support new breastfeeding mothers and infants need for success. WIC State and local agencies are required by WIC Program regulations to create policies and procedures to ensure breastfeeding support and assistance is provided throughout the prenatal and postpartum period, particularly when the mother is most likely to need assistance.

Furthermore, the government has introduced the "Loving Support Award of Excellence" program to recognize those WIC *agencies* that have been shown to provide excellent breastfeeding promotion and support for WIC participants. This award program is intended, in part, to motivate other agencies to strengthen their own programs by increasing breastfeeding rates among mothers receiving WIC monies (United States, 2018). We'd like to emphasize that this award is going to the *agencies* not the individual mothers. While we admit that it is advantageous for mothers at or below the poverty line to receive assistance with breastfeeding, we also note that such programming creates a new form of surveilling the mother who needs governmental support. As you will see in the following WIC documents (see Figures 5.1 and 5.2), there are many rules and restrictions for what new mothers and their babies can receive based upon the degree to which the mother is breastfeeding. From the government, to the local WIC agency, to the local grocery store, financially struggling mothers are now surveilled and rewarded or punished based upon what choices they make in feeding their children.

Once again, we certainly support the premise that women need all the support they can receive to breastfeed their babies—and such a need seems to exist even more so within communities of color and those who are economically disadvantaged. At the same time, the medical-scientific-institutional gaze which we have been discussing turns all mothers into objects of subjection. But, the governmental surveillance that is integral to this particular gaze couldn't be enacted more violently than it is for non-white, non-middle class women. Citing Guibert, Foucault (1995) declares "discipline must be made national" (p. 169)! Such is the case for breastfeeding mothers, in general, and for mothers of color and those who are economically challenged, more specifically. These governmental monitoring policies have become a form of national policing that stand ready to refuse a low-income mother an extra gallon of milk if she isn't breastfeeding. Punishment is indeed a political tactic (Foucault, 1995, p. 23) that serves to benefit and perpetuate the current power structures. By maintaining the gaze on the docile body (the new mother) (Foucault, 1995), larger structures of power do not need to be questioned.

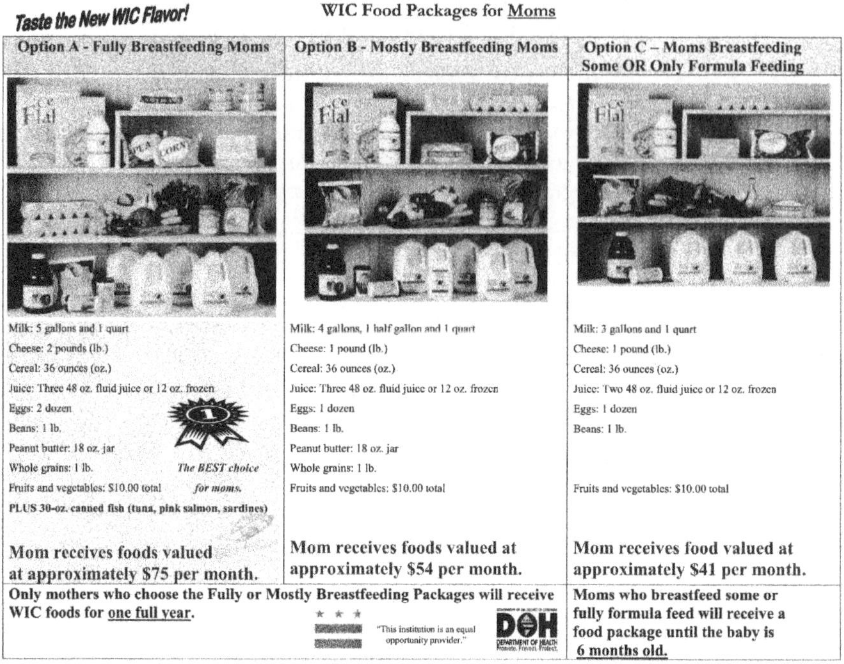

Figure 5.1. WIC Food Packages for Moms. Chart courtesy of the Department of Health/ Pictures courtesy of the WIC Program.

REFRAMING THE QUESTION

Sadly, the current framing of breastfeeding among women of color, and those who are low income and have less education totally ignores structural factors. Given the fact that the ability to take paid time off of work post-partum, to have a job upon return, to have a workplace that allows time and a sanitary, private place for mothers to pump and a refrigerator to store their milk, to have health insurance, and to belong to a social network that supports new parents are pre-requisites to breastfeeding, there can be no doubt that only certain mothers and families are privileged with this lived reality—and by this point in this book, we know who those are. As author Alissa Quart (2012) stated "pumping daily illustrated to me how social class and labor rights are utterly embedded in the breast-feeding discussion. And yet these underlying issues are not often articulated" (n.p.) In other words, the societal and governmental pressures to breastfeeding that focus solely on what is wrong with the mother without carefully and purposefully critiquing the societal barriers that exist, making it easier for some women and harder for others, is

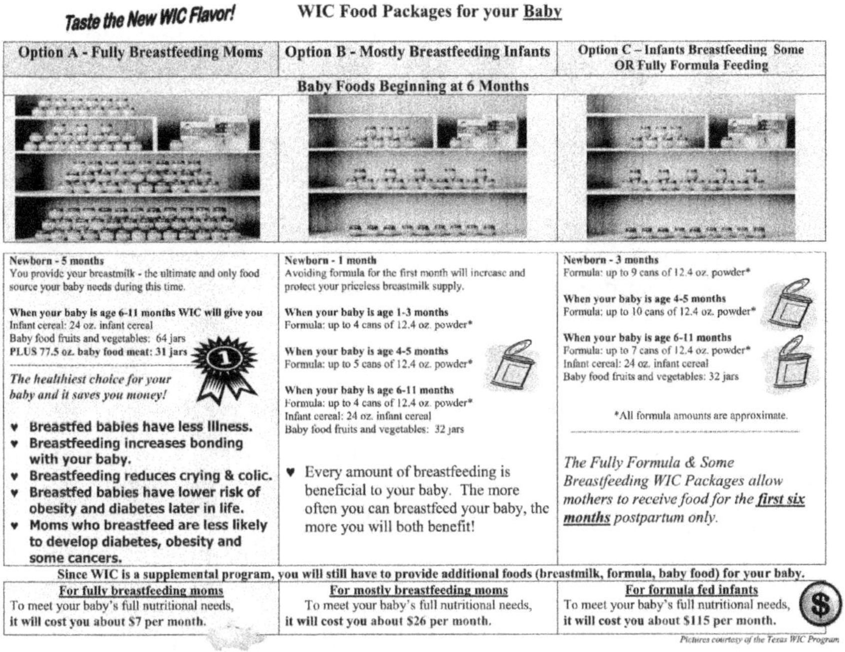

Figure 5.2. WIC Food Packages for Your Baby. Chart courtesy of the Department of Health/ Pictures courtesy of the WIC Program.

another form of structural racism and classism. We agree with Wright and Schanler (2001), who stated

> "while it is 'known' that breastfeeding is better, our society is not structured to facilitate that choice" (Retsinas, 1987). Our efforts to improve breastfeeding rates have to make visible the wider cultural context in which infant feeding choices are made, and alter those components that make it difficult for American women to feed their infants optimally. (p. 424S)

In order to provide all Americans with the same rights to choose how to feed their babies, we must admit that many of the structures embedded within and created by the various breastfeeding discursive formations function as another form of structural racism, heterosexism, and classism. Change cannot happen without a widening of the lens, without questioning these power sources. It is imperative that we broaden the gaze to include governmental agencies, institutions, and workplace, parenting policies, just to name a few. For example, an analysis of the "first food system" conducted by the Center for Social Inclusion (A structural race analysis, 2015) revealed how medical infrastructures, community resources, and employment policies are important interconnected systems that need to be examined together to help change breastfeeding practices. Note how this analysis began with a question about the first food system, a focus on larger societal factors rather than the constant surveilling, monitoring, and quantifying of the mother. Specifically, it is noted that

> This report shows that challenges to breastfeeding are not impossible to overcome. Rather, working together and across the many systems that impact a mother's ability to breastfeed, we can increase rates of breastfeeding for all mothers.
>
> By working to implement the interventions described above, we believe that all mothers and their children will be able to choose breastfeeding and benefit from its physical and psychological advantages, leading to better health outcomes for everyone. (A structural race analysis, 2015, p. 18)

Similar to this analysis, we propose that we need to ask different questions in order to generate different knowledge. For example, rather than ask what barriers exist that prevent mothers of color (etc.) from breastfeeding or what keep women of color from breastfeeding, we need to ask, how can we help all individuals make the feeding choice that is right for them and their family? Or what beliefs, practices, structures have led to Asian and Hispanic women breastfeeding more than any other women? What if we asked what are the *pathways* to fully actualized motherhood? A pathway, in our opinion, that provides a balanced perspective on breast *and* formula feeding; respects all mothers' choices; understands and respects how culture, race, education, income differences among women impact their choice; and provides helpful, realistic information about formula *and* breastfeeding to all mothers and their families. Integral to all of these visions of actualized motherhood are changes to employment laws at local, state, and federal levels that support the needs of new mothers and their families. In addition, we must identify solutions for delivering excellent and affordable child care for all working parents and create a more equitable health care system that serves all women of all backgrounds.

Finally, we must also question the scientific gaze. While many of us tend to accept science and statistics as objective and factual, we want to challenge that assumption. The variable-analytic approach, which we have argued, is similar to the "classifactory gaze" (Foucault, 1994), and "is sensitive only to the surface divisions" (p. 6). As we discussed in this chapter, science is never neutral. Accordingly, it is incumbent upon us to interrogate the biased approach behind these numbers, or to engage in what Foucault (1994) calls "commentary," a process by which we try to "uncover the deeper meaning of speech" (p. xiv). We must ask who are the gatekeepers of knowledge production and dissemination? How do their positions of power influence the type of inquiry conducted and the questions asked? What do they seek to gain from the knowledge created? As already noted, large governmental agencies such as the CDC, HHS, and NIS are charged with tracking breastfeeding rates. They then often disseminate the numbers via governmental documents such as the Surgeon General's Call to Action and to organizations such as WHO and LLLI. This large knowledge production machinery has led to an institutionalization of breastfeeding whereby the breastfeeding mother is at once the patient (Foucault, 1994) and the prisoner (Foucault, 1995)—subjected to both medical and institutionalized gazes.

Even after the decades of pressure appeals by pro-breastfeeding advocates, governmental oversight, international marketing restrictions, baby-friendly hospitals, grant monies paid to universities and research organizations, and global initiatives, thousands and thousands of U.S. women are still resisting the ideological pressures of the breast-is-best paradigm—and most notably, African American mothers. Some may say that is exactly the reason why more pro-breastfeeding advocacy is needed. We say, instead, that this is the reason to reframe the problem.

NOTES

1. Kimberly Seals Allers, Mocha Manual.com: Motherhood in color. Retrieved July 13, 2019 from http://mochamanual.com.
2. Black Mothers Breastfeeding Club of Detroit. Retrieved July 13, 2019 from http://blackmothersbreastfeeding.org/.
3. Salud America, About. Retrieved July 13, 2019 from https://salud-america.org/about/.
4. Mommy's Wall, Online invitations that make gathering easier. Retrieved from http://www.mommyswall.com/.

SIX

Talking Back

The Discourses of Lived Experience

> "Make your own choice. It's really up to you and what you—you think's best for your child."
>
> (Amber, interviewee)

> "Really, in the end, it was myself. As far as it was something that I knew that I was gonna have to decide to do, and my decision was gonna affect me as well as the child."
>
> (Carolina, interviewee)

> ". . . to me it was really my decision, not his because I'm, I'm doing the feeding. And the breast, the milk has to come out of my breast, not his."
>
> (Jenna, interviewee)

> "I don't think the doctor was too happy. But, I mean, it's not their body, it's mine."
>
> (Crystal, interviewee)

These quotes come from several women we have interviewed throughout the years about their breast and bottle-feeding experiences.[1] Up to this point in the book, we have reviewed a variety of pro-breastfeeding discourses that work together to form a tight knot around women's bodies, squeezing away their agentic rights to be the kind of mother they want to be and, in turn, discursively forming the construct we have labeled hegemonic mothering. Figuratively, this knot takes the breath away from countless mothers who choose to formula feed their infants, disciplining them, silencing them and, in some instances, erasing their full personhood. You will notice embedded in the women's stories references to the omnipotent forms of power and knowledge, surveilling and punishing them when not following what is natural—breastfeeding their child. In this chapter, it is the mothers' turn to talk back to this form of hegemonic mothering and our turn to listen. We have heard many stories from our interviewees, acquaintances, friends, and family members about how they were pressured to breastfeed and how this form of hegemonic mothering left many in tears, feeling despair and helplessness. Sadly, these stories are far too common. As you will soon read, many experienced extreme anxiety as they fought the societal forces telling them that breast was THE only way to mother. You will also hear stories of resiliency and how many of these same mothers broke through the societal, medical, and familial ideological knots that were silencing them. We see the stories shared herein as a form of discursive resistance—a way for these women to speak as subjects to their own lived experiences and break free from the binds that tie them to hegemonic motherhood. We invite you to listen to these women; to really feel the emotions between the lines.

We start with Sarah.[2]

SARAH'S STORY

I look back and feel like I was a child bride at the tender age of 25. My husband and I eloped in Las Vegas and about as quickly as we decided to get married, we decided to get pregnant about 9 months after the wedding. We were young, spontaneous, and dumb. We got pregnant after my birthday weekend in Charleston and—not knowing it was already too late—decided after that weekend we were not ready to be parents and decided to continue using protection.

But it is true what they say, it can really only take one time (or weekend in our case). We were excited and nervous. But secretly, I felt very alone. None of my friends were pregnant or married or anywhere near that stage of their life. I was about to venture in a world of the unknown with no friends, no directions and even though I had my husband it still wasn't enough.

I also wasn't your typical "mother to be." I did not like seeing my body changing. I did not think pregnancy was beautiful. I read the books but still ate soft cheese because "my mother did." I did not want to do Lamaze classes. I did not want to see *The Miracle of Birth*. I didn't want a tour of the hospital. I did not want a mirror during my labor to watch the baby come out (ew gross) and I did not want to breastfeed. What is funny is that I managed to escape all of the above except the breastfeeding. When asked to write this story it came easy because I felt a tremendous amount of pressure to breastfeed. Not just by our culture but by our health care providers. I will say it—I truly detested the breastfeeding consultant. What are they called "lactation specialists?" They acted as if any other option was selfish and insane. "Breast is best" after all (insert eye roll).

So, when I had my first son, I gave it a go even though my own mother said "the hell with them, just bottle feed. That's what I did, and you all came out fine." This is one of the many times I should have listened to my mother, but as a first-time mother, I wanted to do everything right and at that moment I didn't want to disappoint anyone. I wanted to be perfect and give the best to my baby. Now in reflection, I know that this is silly because everything I have learned about motherhood is anything but perfection.

But still, I gave it a go. The old college try! The minute Tobyn was born he was laid on my chest, the nurses moved the paper-like night gown to bare my naked breast (which honestly embarrassed me to have the entire room see my gigantic breasts) and guided Tobyn towards it. He tried to latch and was unsuccessful.

A failure already and just minutes after birth, what a moment! I just did one of the most amazing things a body can do and already I failed. The nurses assured me of course that he would latch. They brought in lactation consultants and continued to force him to my breast. I had more women feel my breasts in 48 hours than men in my high school years, and I loathed it.

But finally, on the third day my milk came in, he finally latched consistently and then he never left it. To say I hated breastfeeding was an understatement. My breasts were so large, they did not have a bra to fit me at the maternity store. I had so much milk, I would wake up in the middle of the night with my sheets soaked. I could have been a wet nurse. I had breast milk stocked for days. In my mind, I kept saying just make it to 6 weeks, it is only 6 weeks! I knew all the research; 6 weeks is best for the baby—it is most important to his development, breastfed babies are smarter and healthier, blah blah blah. I continued to struggle and during the 4th week I had a hole in my nipple the size of a pea and was making pink milk from the constant bleeding. I called the doctor immediately thinking, this could not be healthy for the baby secretly hoping it wasn't and I could stop breastfeeding. But of course, the nurse assured me the baby would be fine and the nipples would "toughen up" in time. In the end, I developed mastitis which is an infection in your breast that causes flu-like symptoms. When I called about this and scheduled an appointment, I was told to continue breastfeeding. I walked out of the office and bought formula on the way home cursing them. I started the horrific process of weaning the next day.

When I stopped breastfeeding I found myself making excuses with anyone who asked my why I stopped. I would lie and extend the amount of time I breastfed to make the six week cut off so at least I could say "I made it six weeks which as we know from research is the most pivotal time for the baby" or "breastfeeding was harder than birth for me." Yes, I lied. I lied because I didn't want the judgment. I made it 5 weeks and guess what? Tobyn is in all advanced classes, healthy, athletic, and has never had any issues with development.

You would think I would have learned my lesson with my second child but I tried again in the hopes that my first attempt was a fluke. The same thing happened with Cooper, and I weaned at 4 weeks. He is also in all of the advanced classes and healthy as a horse.

DEAR MOM FRIENDS

By Kristen

I am a white, middle class married female with four children. The journey to have four children was riddled with fertility issues, numerous doctors' appointments, treatments, procedures, fertility drugs, and failed attempts. I was the "this is so interesting, we've never seen this before" patient. It was a daunting process, but that story is for another time.

When we finally got pregnant with our first child, William, we felt like it was a miracle and at the time, felt like having one was all we needed, especially with all we had been through. I will never forget my mother's excitement that we were pregnant, but it quickly followed with "are you going to breastfeed?" You ARE going to breastfeed right?" This comment didn't surprise me in the least bit. My mother took great pride in breastfeeding and when I say great pride I mean this was something she shared with EVERYONE. She felt like breastfeeding was the reason I didn't have allergies, why I have "beautiful skin" and everything in between. Breastfeeding was and still is, as crazy as it might sound, her greatest pride as a mother. I worried about breastfeeding William before he even arrived. I worried if I would produce enough milk, I worried about everything. I went to a breastfeeding class where I felt like mothers, some second time mothers, knew much more than I did already. I remember hearing from my doctor, the lactation consultant and what felt like everyone else, how great breastfeeding is and how bad formula was. I left the breastfeeding class with a folder of all its benefits. I thought, at that time, why would I now breastfeed? When William was born and I was in the hospital, I remember being asked if I wanted him to stay with me for the night or in the nursery. Before I had a chance to answer, the nurse said, "oh, if you are breastfeeding he has to stay with you." I was SO tired; I wanted to rest. Immediately, I felt like this whole breastfeeding thing wasn't going to feel as natural as it should. I already felt completely consumed by it, but it got much worse. My milk finally came in and this was after massaging my breasts and pumping with the hospital pump to stimulate the breasts to produce milk. Before I could breastfeed on my own, I needed help. They began supplementing with formula only because my milk hadn't come in yet, but they didn't want him to have too much formula so that he could get as much as he could get from breast milk. They sent us home with formula, but not much. They didn't want me to give up on breastfeeding. I still wasn't producing milk like I felt like I should be. I was struggling. I was struggling mentally more than physically. WHY wasn't I producing lots of milk, why was this so hard, why could my mom do this AND enjoy it and I couldn't. It was very frustrating. I would text with close friends about breastfeeding, seeking advice and asking questions. Finally, I decided to reach out to the lactation consultant at the hospital; I took William with me. She asked me to show her how he latched on and after trying a few times he finally latched on correctly. He fed for maybe 30 seconds and then stopped. She was happy to see that he could do it but after mashing my boob into his mouth several times to do it again she pulled out a plastic nipple shield and let me try it. It was like putting a bottle nipple on your nipple. It was amazing at first. It worked! After leaving, with the understanding that I should use that if I need it, but not to let him get too use to it, and breastfeeding should get better as he pulled my nipple out. It was never confirmed I had inverted nipples, but that's what the nipple shield was used for, as I was told. We went home and I was optimistic. A few days later after using the nipple shield almost solely, because it worked for William and me, I still wasn't producing enough milk to sustain him. I went back to the lactation consultant and she gave me a contraption that has a long skinny tube you clip on to your bra and out of that skinny tube comes formula so as the baby is sucking your nipple he is getting food through the tube. I suppose this makes the baby want to suck more and it also stimulates milk production for me. It was a milky mess. At this point my husband saw my frustration and told me it was "ok" if I didn't want to breastfeed anymore. He was so great about it, but I was determined. I decided I was going to pump and we would just bottle feed with breast milk I pumped. I did this for about two months when everything took a turn. I was in the shower one night and I heard William crying with my husband. I was enjoying my hot shower and was trying to ignore the crying. My husband had a long day at work and the crying was getting to him. I yelled from the shower that he was probably hungry and I would feed him when I got out and as he continued to cry, I could tell my husband was getting more and more frustrated. Finally, he yelled, "I don't know what to do" and I ripped open the shower curtain and grabbed towel and said "give him to me!" and I walked in the kitchen, fixed a bottle of formula and said "HERE!" I got back in the shower and started to cry. I couldn't handle it anymore. I was the sole "feeder" of William and I hated it. I am an independent woman and I can't stand to think that I am obligated to something that I didn't feel like I had control over. Breastfeeding was controlling me and it wasn't going well and I hated it. It wasn't the bonding experience for William and me that I was told it would be, and it wasn't easy or natural for me. This was my breaking point. From then on, my mom encouraged me to keep trying, not to give up after nights and nights of waking up soaked in milk I decided I was done. William was about 3 months old when I transitioned him solely to formula. I cried to my doctor and my OB/GYN about this. My doctor was surprisingly great and seeing my distress said, "as long as babies get fed one way or the other, they will be fine" and I felt like saying, "where was this person when I was trying to decide to breastfeed or not?" I found out that many, many people had the same experience as I did, but not until after the struggle, after beating myself up and after blaming myself for not trying hard enough or long enough. It was a HUGE relief to formula feed. Yes, it was more expensive, but it was well worth it. Anyone could feed William, I didn't have to worry about needing to feed him because my breasts felt like they were going to burst (when they were full of milk), and I could leave him with anyone and I didn't have to make time to pump at work, etc.; it was a HUGE burden lifted.

I did try to breastfeed my second child, Bray, but it went the same way. I told myself I wouldn't feel guilty about not breastfeeding, but I did. I almost felt worse with him. I did go through postpartum depression with him, which was very hard. I tried for maybe 2 months with Bray and then decided to go with formula. I didn't catch as much grief for not breastfeeding him because everyone knew I had stopped with William. My mother never let me forget that I didn't breastfeed.

For quite some time the decision to not breastfeed haunted me. Not breastfeeding made me feel like I wasn't doing what was best for my children; that they weren't getting "natural" nutrients. After sharing my story with others who were quick to tell me not to be so hard on myself, I eventually felt like my transition to formula was what was best for me—emotionally—and was just fine for my kids. It wasn't until my twins arrived (my last children) that I knew going into my appointments and even the hospital that I was going to stand firm and let them know that I might not breastfeed. I decided to be open to it and see how things went in the hospital so that the babies could get the colostrum, at the very minimum, but I quickly let the nurses and doctors know that I had struggled with my others and while I was aware of the benefits it was too hard on me emotionally to try with TWO! It took a very long time to gain the balls to stand my ground and be OK with formula feeding.

JESSICA'S WORDS

My insecurities with breastfeeding likely began decades before I became pregnant with my first child. My twelve-year-old prayers (more like pleading) for my breasts to stop growing, proved unnecessary. Ironically my "flatness" earned me the affectionate nickname of "chest" for the remainder of my high school days.

My chest size certainly wasn't the only reason I doubted my ability to breastfeed. There was the ever-present fact that I was diagnosed with Leukemia as a young child and my body had already gone through cocktails of chemotherapy. With severe generalized anxiety, I was constantly aware that my current medication "could" be passed on to my child through breast milk. These are just a few of the reasons that I wasn't completely confident that I could fulfill the traditional image of the serene and nurturing female figure providing pure and natural sustenance for a helpless human.

Through the pregnancy, surprisingly I didn't really focus that much on breastfeeding. I didn't need to as it was presented to me as the ideal way to raise your child. I have always been a bit of a perfectionist so ideal was a great place to land. Combined with my perfectionism is a healthy dose of realism and acceptance that the experience is all part of the process. I've taught myself to reject the "white picket fences" narrative. I think these two perspectives combined are what drove my answer to the frequent question, "Are you planning to breastfeed?." I don't ever remember confidently saying "yes." Instead, the response was almost always, "we're gonna give it a shot."

My birth plan was always, "get the baby out in a way that is safe for me and him." I trusted the doctors and nurses to make the decisions from there. Because I had to be induced on my due date because of high blood pressure, the whole idea of a delivery being "natural" quickly became subjective.

My son was born at 5:36 PM on a Monday. By Tuesday night he was screaming constantly and I was crying constantly. Of course we had been working regularly to teach him to latch and start to feed, but it was obvious that he wasn't getting enough—if anything at all. He was hungry; I knew that was natural. My husband and I talked about what to do. I knew the "risks" of giving my son anything but the breast. How could I NOT know the risks? I ran through the scenarios in my head and somehow the realist in me managed to win and remind me that the child was hungry. He needed food. He wasn't getting it from me. Decision made. I signed the forms to allow the nurses to give my son a bottle. *Yes, I know "breast is best"; Yes, I know this is not what is recommended; Yes, now please give him some food!* He took several ounces from the bottle immediately and fell asleep.

I honestly don't remember much about the first month at home with my son. Mentally I was completely overwhelmed and exhausted. Physically I was okay, but mentally I did not believe this. The breastfeeding (with a bottle supplement here and there) became the normal routine. My mental state was anything but normal and routine. I was afraid to sleep for fear that I might not wake up; I was afraid to sleep for fear that the baby might not wake up. I remember my husband attempting to revive my interest in the sitcom *Wings*. To this day I can't watch that show without feeling panic rise from my stomach.

I should mention that during the pregnancy and after, I had been advised to decrease my medicinal dosage quite a bit. A month after giving birth I had to face one of those "realistic" decisions. It was clear by that point I needed to take something to help me cope with the mental effects of having a child. The challenge: If I increased my medicine or changed medicine, I would have to stop breastfeeding. If I stop breastfeeding, the chances are slim that I could start again. In many ways, I believed I had failed. This wasn't ideal. I had given up on breastfeeding my child after a month and not because "it wasn't working" but because "I wasn't working." I was selfishly prioritizing my health over the baby's. But I needed help and needed it fast. Decision made—we would stop breastfeeding. I gave myself a month to recover mentally.

For one month, I pumped several times a day and dumped the milk down the drain.

Despite the "warnings" my son was very flexible and easily moved between the breast and the bottle. This allowed me to jump back into the breastfeeding game as soon as I had gotten my emotional state under control and the medicine was "safe" for the baby. We continued our routine of breastfeeding and bottle feeding. I tried the herbal supplements. I tried the extra pumping. I just never had enough and that had to be okay. By month three of life (really only month two of breastfeeding) my son was taking two bottles of breast milk a day while I worked, eating from me 2 to 3 times a day when I was home, and taking formula to supplement everything in between. It worked.

When my son approached 9 months of age, he began showing signs of being disinterested in eating from the breast. It was so much easier for him (and easier for me) to take the bottles. It was okay. It had to be. We were done. I did find myself justifying the fact that it was ONLY 9 months of breastfeeding on several occasions. I constantly justified the supplementing. I usually didn't share the fact that he had really only fed from me for 8 months. Eight months was good enough right? I had friends that didn't even try to breastfeed so I had to get points for trying—right? I knew it wasn't the recommended first year of life, but it was close. When asked if I breastfed the answer became, "well, yeah for like 9 months. We did supplement some because I just didn't have enough." I cringed a little every time I shared. Did I try hard enough? Did I give up too soon? Was it enough to see benefits?

Three years after the birth of my first son, my second son made his appearance. I used the same lines—"we're gonna try." My expectations were low and honestly for one of the first times in my life, I was totally okay with that. Like many stressful aspects of life, once you let go of the pressure sometimes things fall into place. My second son easily latched and was exclusively breastfed for two months. We started supplementing with a small bottle to help him sleep around month three because . . . well, why not? He was hungry and we all needed sleep. At 12 months my youngest became more interested in socializing with the outside world and less interested in eating from me; I remember realizing that "we made it."

I would love to say that I had some profound insights on the long-term benefits or drawbacks of breastfeeding, but I don't. Ironically, while my husband, my youngest son, and I were almost exclusively breastfed, my oldest son (was breastfed the least) is by far the most physically healthy member of our family. My youngest has always desired more physical connection with me but I don't know if that is in any way related to our "success" with the breastfeeding.

For the perfectionist in me, not trying was not an option. I appreciate the experiences that the drive has given me. I am equally thankful for the realist voices that prompted my decisions to go with what worked and was most logical. Breastfeeding security and confidence is not something I ever achieved. I now know that it is not something that I ever needed.

KAREN'S TALE

I'm white, 35 year old, hold a master's degree, and am in the middle class. I had 2 pretty normal pregnancies that were 7 years apart.

I was told with my first pregnancy that I needed to breastfeed because it was best for the baby. I only breastfed my first for about 8 weeks, and the whole time felt frustrated, tired, and not quite like a mom because I wasn't producing milk like I thought I would. I decided to switch to formula, and felt bad about it and that I had failed my baby. Of course, he was fine, and slept better, cried less, and we were both happier! But still felt like I failed him in some way.

With my 2nd pregnancy, I was determined to breastfeed longer. I had a girlfriend who is my age, and she breastfed her babies until they were 2. So I felt some pressure that I had to breastfeed longer. This one I tried pumping as much as I could, taking lactation cookies, and I still wasn't producing enough. I remember crying to my husband that I felt like a failure again as a mom because I wasn't enough for my baby. But he was supportive and encouraged me that it was okay. He actually begged me to give him formula because our baby was cranky, upset, and obviously hungry.

I felt like I was a failure because I could only breastfeed for a couple of months, and had to switch to formula afterwards. My mom was supportive, my husband was supportive, but I did feel like my friend was judging me because I didn't try everything I could (supplements) to keep up my milk production.

I just wish everyone didn't have an opinion on what you "should" do for YOUR baby! We're all moms. We're all just doing our best!

KATIE, M.ED., 36, WHITE FEMALE

I got pregnant with my first son, Auggie, in 2013. My pregnancy was pretty typical, and I had no issues or complications so I spent most of my time focusing on childbirth and parenting. In 2004 I had a breast reduction, so I knew I would have a hard time breastfeeding. In fact, the doctor who performed the surgery made sure that I knew about the possibility that I would not be able to breastfeed before I would agree to move forward with the procedure. I told myself at the beginning of my pregnancy that it wasn't a big deal and I would do what I could, but it was ok if I needed to formula feed and my husband agreed to support me with whatever was best for me and our child. However, throughout my pregnancy, I did what most pregnant millennial parents do and I read a bunch of parenting books and blogs. I read a lot about breastfeeding vs formula feeding and eventually become convinced that I needed to try as hard as I could to breastfeed. Everything I read pointed to unbelievable benefits of breastfeeding. It started to feel as if anything less than breastfeeding for at least a year could harm my child emotionally and physically. In addition to what I was reading, everyone around me asked if I planned to breastfeed my child. If I made the mistake of saying no or I wasn't sure, folks made sure to let me know about all the benefits of breastfeeding. I was told by more than one parent that I would regret not breastfeeding because I wouldn't have that "special bond" with my son. If that didn't work, folks would remind me that breastfeeding would help me lose the baby weight because shaming a new mom's body is apparently a last ditch effort to make women feel motivated enough to breastfeed at all costs.

About 6 months into my pregnancy, I bought the book, *Defining Your Own Success: Breastfeeding After Breast Reduction Surgery*. The book had great advice for those that wanted to breastfeed after a reduction and I learned about new resources available for parents including nipple shields, ways to hold your baby, pumping and feeding schedules, etc. The book also had stories of women who chose to breastfeed after a reduction. A pattern within the stories started to emerge for me. Most of the women stated that they wish they had not made the "selfish" decision to have a breast reduction because it could prevent them from giving their child the very best they have to offer. It could cause their child to be sicker, less emotionally connected, and have less educational opportunities. At one point, I put the book down and never picked it back up because I felt ashamed every time I read it.

Around the same time, my husband and I went to new parent meetings with pediatricians to choose a doctor for our son. At one doctor's office, the nurse took the first 10 minutes to discuss the importance of breastfeeding. She asked if everyone in the room planned to breastfeed. Not wanting to have to explain myself, I said yes as did everyone else. She let out a huge sigh and said, "thank goodness." She told us that parents who breastfed their children had smaller medical files than the children who were formula fed. She went on to talk about how sick the formula fed kids were and that she preferred to work with breastfed kids because they were "easier." We did not choose that doctor and I left their office crying.

While my pregnancy was uneventful, childbirth was another story. After several complications, 24 hours of labor, an epidural that didn't work, and a vacuum birth as the result of a 9lb 7oz baby with the head size above the 100th percentile, I was exhausted and somewhat traumatized. I was in the hospital for five days due to both mine and my son's complications and in that time, I tried to breastfeed. However, given the fact that my son was over 9lbs and my history with the breast reduction, breastfeeding was not going well. The nurses were incredibly helpful and empathetic. However, at one point a nurse grabbed my breast to help produce milk. She squeezed so hard that I just started crying. My husband gave my son his first bottle of formula in the hospital and I remember feeling like I had failed. I limited the amount of formula I would allow my son to get because I was afraid of nipple confusion and a preference for formula over breast milk.

After we left the hospital, I tried everything I could to get breast milk for my son. He would feed for about an hour and a half and an hour later I would try to pump. I was attached to my son or a pump for the first few weeks at home. I spent lots of money on a hospital grade pump, fenugreek pills, lactation cookies, nipple shields, and pumping supplies and bras. I was awake all the time and my son didn't get enough to eat so he cried nonstop. My nipples and breasts hurt from the nonstop feeding and pumping and every time I put my son to my breast I would yell from the pain. I started to resent my son, my husband, and being a parent in general. I was miserable.

One morning, about two weeks after bringing our son home, I woke up rested but, in a panic, because my son wasn't making any noises even though I did not wake up for his midnight feeding. My husband fed him formula overnight so that I could sleep. He got a chance to bond with our son and I got my first full night of sleep in weeks. I remember feeling guilty that I had slept and taken care of myself. In my mind, parenting was about making incredible sacrifices for my children. Even the small act of getting sleep for the night meant I wasn't doing everything in my power to do the best for my child. However, even given all those feelings, I was rested and felt more like myself and my son was sleeping because he was no longer starving. We made the decision to formula feed and I would slowly wean him off breastfeeding in time for me to go back to work. I started bonding with my son and husband and I was able to get out of the house because I no longer had a pump attached to my breasts. Everything got a lot easier after we made the decision to formula feed. I still got a few reactions and dirty looks from other parents whenever I would shake up my powder formula for him but we knew we were doing what was best for everyone in our family and I just choose my mom friends wisely. When my second son was born we started with formula from day one so we wouldn't have the same experience as the first time. It changed my relationship with my son and my husband and I had my body back.

EXCEPT IT DIDN'T

BY JENNI

My water broke around 9:00pm on September 29th, 2010. I will never forget my husband, standing in our bedroom in his old, ripped jeans, looking at me incredulously. "Why aren't you more nervous?" he asked/demanded.

"What should I be nervous about?" I'd really thought this. I really asked it. This was the most natural thing in the world. I'd never felt more in control. More calm. My water broke. There was no guess work. Yes. I was in labor. My body knew what to do.

Except, it didn't. My water had broken, but my baby was sitting tight (I find this to be a character trait with this particular child . . .). At 9:00am the next morning, my doctor decided to induce. Keenan came a few hours later. He was perfect. He had my beloved grandmother's blue eyes, adorable lips, and a perfect nose. I had barely looked at him before the nurse asked me if I was breastfeeding. The question was almost immediate.

I responded with a resounding, "yes." I mean, of course I was going to breastfeed. All of the books I'd read, all of the online forums I'd perused—everything—had told me to breastfeed. Nothing had ever really said how that was done (or what to do if you didn't), but this was nature. It would all work out. The nurse gave me a look of approval and said, "Yes! That's what we like to hear." So, only a few minutes in and I was killing this mom thing. Everything was working out.

Except it wasn't and didn't. It just seemed like it in the imaginary world I'd created by endlessly preparing myself for this moment. Keenan latched on immediately. He knew what to do and I followed his lead. Things seemed to be going wonderfully. Keenan cried a lot, but he was a newborn. I'd read my books. I knew that was normal. He lost a little weight, but that was expected—my books said so. We were discharged and took our sweet baby home.

Two days later, we met with the pediatrician. Keenan was turning yellow. He wouldn't stop crying. He wasn't having dirty diapers. He'd lost too much weight between birth and the appointment. Things were bad. They were really, really bad.

Because I had been induced, my milk wasn't letting down. The medicine used to induce expecting mothers effects the way their milk lets down. At least that was what I was told at this appointment. But never before that.

Keenan was starving. My baby was starving. My pediatrician sent me home with some formula. I hadn't bought any. My books specifically said I didn't need to. I had all the food my baby needed. They told me that!

Except, I didn't. I was devastated. The pediatrician looked at me with a smile and said, "Some mothers never produce enough milk. I don't know what happened to babies before formula. They probably died."

In reality, some survived, some didn't. I know that now. I know that the formula I was given was making my baby better. My milk did eventually let down, but I never produced enough of it to feed Keenan exclusively. In addition, Keenan's esophagus hadn't fully developed which meant he had trouble keeping milk down. He was called a "happy spitter" (but he wasn't very happy) and would be one until he started eating solid foods.

Because he had trouble with feeding, every mother I knew tried to "show" me how to do it. How *they* could do it. "Jenni, if you just make him take breaks," "if you just use this bottle instead of that one . . . " I felt so inadequate. Except when Keenan spit up all over them after they'd shown me "how to do it." Then I felt vindicated! I loved my son so much in those moments! I relished explaining to them—again—what a happy spitter was.

But in reality, it was really hard. I worried so much for Keenan. Sometimes . . . I was afraid of him. I couldn't do anything right and I thought I was breaking him. It started with the breastfeeding and lack there of. Sometimes I would wonder, "If I knew inducing affected milk supply, would I have been induced?" Honestly, I had these questions and concerns until Keenan started eating solid foods.

I have two healthy sons now and I have the benefit of retrospect. My kids are fine. They always were because I live in a developed country with safe drinking water and access to formula. I never produced enough milk to feed either of them exclusively, but where Keenan made it to three months on my milk and formula, Reece made to eight months. No issues, good eater. No worries. I got sick at eight months and had to wean him, but I was confident I'd done my job. It was an entirely different experience the second time around. As I write this, they seem to have the same intelligence, or perhaps, decision-making skills—they make equally bad ones, especially when together! They get sick about the same as their peers—sometimes less, sometimes more. They. Are. Thriving.

I asked Danny, my husband, to write something for this. He didn't want to. He said, "I don't know what to say. I just felt bad for you." The whole time he knew it would be fine, but I'd been so indoctrinated into "The Breast Is Exclusive," I couldn't see out of it. I'm drawn to the "Father Knows Best" section of *What to Expect When You're Expecting.* What if he had read that? What if he had thought I was doing something wrong, too. I don't know what I would have done. I would have been alone . . . and poor Keenan. It breaks my heart thinking about it.

STOP THE JUDGMENT, PLEASE!

By Loreen

I said "no; I am not going to breastfeed.
I am having twins
and I want my husband to be an equal partner in their care.
I don't need to breastfeed to bond with my baby."
I know enough about science to understand the bias inherent in the breastfeeding research.
I know countless people, myself included, who were formula fed, and we turned out just fine.
No. I am not going to breastfeed.
Until, they were born.
I said "sure. I'll try."
I gave in to the pressure.
I had a c-section and a difficult recovery.
Nurses said babies were fine. Momma needed to heal.
Babies were given formula.
Momma said okay; I was in too much pain to do anything different.
I recovered; my babies were combo-fed.
One baby was a "lazy eater," the other was very easy to breastfeed.
I have tubes taped all over my breasts, so it is easier for my struggling baby to eat,
but he's still losing weight.
Lactation consultant tells me to breastfeed exclusively to prevent nipple confusion.
My baby is still not eating enough. I must supplement.
I am failing as a mom.
What are these big boobs for if not to give my babies sustenance?
I can't do this anymore.

I am crying; my husband is trying to console me; my mother is rocking babies.
No more!
I am done trying to live up to some ideal that isn't real.
Give these babies a bottle; give me a break!
They are healthy and bright. What more could a mother ask for?
But, why must I explain and justify my decision?
Why must I feel that my reason for ceasing to breastfeed isn't sufficient enough?
Please stop the judgment!
Stop keeping information away from women.
Allow us to exercise our power to make informed decisions that are best for us, our babies, our families, and our bodies.

> "I don't feel right in giving advice whether to breast-feed or not because I really feel that is just a personal decision you have to make."
>
> (E, interviewee)

> " . . . my advice would definitely be that it is okay to um, bottle-feed. That you know, just because they say the "breast is best" doesn't mean it's best for you."
>
> (Jenna, interviewee)

DUAL GENDERED EXPECTATIONS

We have purposely presented these words, reflections—*emotions*—in their original form and let them flow from one woman to the next to let their stories simply *be*. Because what they are *is enough*. These women *are enough*. They are amazing, strong, and capable. Many of these women have become friends and colleagues over the years. Their confidence abounds in so many varied situations and settings. And yet, here they were, talking to us about how inadequate they felt when breastfeeding. Often, women we spoke with were eager to share their stories, because in this one thing, they were so helpless. The language of their stories reveals "the oppressed struggle in language to recover ourselves—to rewrite, to reconcile, to renew. Our words are not without meaning. They are an action—a resistance" (hooks, 2015, p. 28). For these women, and many others, sharing their breastfeeding resistance stories are ways to rewrite motherhood in their own terms.

Moreover, what we see and feel through these narratives is the lived experience of the "double entanglement" (McRobbie, 2009, p. 12) of a sex-gender system that requires women to be all in, all the time. Kristen's account stands out here: "I couldn't handle it anymore. I was the sole 'feeder' of William and I hated it. I am an independent woman and I can't stand to think that I am obligated to something that I didn't feel like I had control over."

The double entanglement of our sex-gender system reveals how "different normative ideas compete with each other. Women are now meant to work like men, but at the same time must always be able to be all women if that is required" (Woltersdor, 2011, p. 173). When it comes to mothering, and as we see through these narratives, particularly breastfeeding, we are required to work harder than men, because what we are doing is the most important thing *we will ever do.*

There are other voices, of course, challenging the institutional narratives controlling these mothers. Sarah's mom, for instance, telling her "the hell with them just bottle feed. That's what I did and you all came out fine," echoes in our minds as we hear Sarah mimicking her mother, who has since passed. But these resistive voices, no matter how strong and influential to the mothers who are speaking, are quieted by the larger institutional discourses that silence them via constant judgment and discipline. So strong are hegemonic discourses maintaining our sex-gender system, that "in the division of labour, in the politics of the family, and in advertisement, traditional ideas of roles are still as dominant as ever" (Woltersdor, 2011, p. 173). These stories are evidence of other arguments we have presented in this book. They are the result of unequal distributions of labor and work, political conservatism, and capitalist commercialism. We are, as Woltersdor (2011) suggests, "still a long way from realizing a freely chosen (and chooseable) neo-gender that would disrupt the hierarchical division into two genders" (p. 173). While hegemonic mothering narratives are meant to empower, they can end up reinforcing patriarchal power structures:

The narratives collected in this chapter show the interconnectedness of hegemonic mothering narratives and how they tie into larger cultural narratives that discipline women. What strikes us most is that in each narrative, save one, we all were afraid to "say no." We were afraid of displeasing the institutional actors perpetuating the narrative and focusing the gaze on our bodies. So, like in so many other situations, we said yes. We gave up our bodies, our autonomy, because we were good girls. Like Jessica, we all wanted to be perfect, because that's what good girls do. The gaze of hegemonic motherhood flows from other narratives that discipline women, telling us to give over our bodies without complaint. As we see with these women, these discourses constrain women. They fail to recognize our full humanness, our abilities to control our own bodies. Loreen's words echo through our heads as we write this book . . . I. Said. No.

NOTES

1. IRB approval was granted by our institution to conduct these interviews. All those identified as "interviewees" were part of this research project and chose their own pseudonyms by which to be identified.

2. The stories presented here were written by family, friends, and acquaintances. Each woman chose a name by which to be identified.

SEVEN

Talking Back and Taking Back

Discourses of Resistance and Change

> Millions of American moms have been "bombarded by a powerful message: that she is built to build a human, that she will feel all the more empowered for doing so as nature supposedly intended and that the baby's future depends on it. Call it the Goddess Myth, spun with a little help from basically everyone—doctors, activists, other moms. It tells us that breast-is-best . . . that your body is a temple and what you put in it should be holy; that sending your baby to the hospital nursery for a few hours after giving birth is a dereliction of duty. Oh, and that you will feel—and look—radiant."
>
> (Howorth, 2017, p. 38)

The words of journalist, Claire Howorth, quoted above capture the state of motherhood in U.S. society. As we have discussed in this book, various discourses and related policies and initiatives have worked together to create a breast-is-best discursive formation. This discursive formation contains, maintains, and perpetuates a certain kind of knowledge—one that privileges exclusive breastfeeding. Power exists within it and is promulgated by that discourse and knowledge, which affords certain entities the ability to set the rules, monitor the subjects (mothers), and punish them when disobeying. Discourses related to intensive mothering, new momism, and total womanhood interact with the breast-is-best discourse reviewed herein. Yet, we argue that the force contained in our discursive formation leads to what we have termed *hegemonic motherhood*. This is a type of motherhood wherein women are expected to put the needs of their children ahead of their own, especially when it comes to breastfeeding. To be a good woman and an excellent mother, one must give birth and breastfeed the baby immediately after delivering her. It is the natural thing to do after all. Your breasts are no longer your own; to declare them off limits to your baby is an act of tyranny—or betrayal. It doesn't matter if you were a rape victim so the touch of your breast by another can be retraumatizing. You're told—get over it! Feeding your baby in this way will be a completely different experience. Not! It doesn't matter if you can't provide enough milk for your baby, and he cries all the time—just keep trying—try harder. With this loss of control over their bodies, mothers' breasts are ripped away from their bodies and turned into objects for others to monitor, to touch, to surveil. This ethos is at the heart of hegemonic mothering—a form of mothering that is shaped by the breast-is-best discursive formation, which serves as a powerful social force *demanding* maternal compliance to the breast-is-best ideology by way of a system of surveillance and punishment. Hegemonic mothering involves the expectation that breastfeeding is an additional way in which mothers' lives are to be devoted to elevating the needs of their children while they suppress their own. This devotion demands that they submit their breasts to the baby who takes ownership of them. The mother's job, above all else, is to keep this liquid gold safe. Society, medical authorities, other moms, and many others surveil mothers and punish them when not complying. As we've heard in this book, mothers who do not are publicly shamed and privately guilt-laden for not abiding by this holy act.

Hegemonic mothering is the result of a variety of discourses that have been structured and ordered in such a way that they cohere around one shared ideology: breast milk is the only acceptable form of infant nutrition. The discourses of medicalization and institutionalization, the discourses of race, class, and privilege, and the discourse of lived experiences discourses, for example, represent interdependent networks, structures, or "orders of discourse" (Fairclough, 1989; Foucault, 1984) with which have worked together to form what we have labeled the Breast-is-Best discursive formation. Importantly, Fairclough (1989) reminds us that "the way in which orders of discourse are structured, and the ideologies which they embody, are determined by relationships of power in particular social institutions, and in the society as a whole" (p. 31). It is society as a whole and certain institutions that have the power to control what mothers do with their bodies and how they feed their babies.

But, there is a resistance growing!

We've argued that the current dominant discourse has swayed in the direction of exclusive breastfeeding. As we draw this book to a close, we look at current resistive discourses to that rhetoric in the form of websites, online bloggers, and social media accounts. We are excited to demonstrate the strong feminist discourses that permeate these artifacts and offer proof that a number of women agree with the aim of this book: to end women vs. women, mother vs. mother rhetorics, and to spread, support, and uphold rhetorics that empower women's autonomy and embrace the choices that we make.

The resistive groups we examine, are perhaps more accurately described as "empowerment groups." They are in conversation with each other in that they seek to create spaces for women who live outside the boundaries of the white, medi-institutionalized discursive formations that shape the realities of breastfeeding. They are not necessarily a coordinated social movement group. Rather, they are independent (mostly) bloggers, who interact with each other in online formats. In that sense, these empowerment groups function along the lines of McGee's (1983) theories of fragmentation. What they lack in formal coordination, they make up for by "following" one another online and by sharing information across platforms. By and large, they function on their own, as disparate texts, that when brought together demonstrate a willingness and desire to change discursive formations of motherhood from dialectical opposites seeking to control, to more open, real, and supportive discourses that seek to empower. So, while they are not (for the most part) formal organizations acting in resistance to dominant narratives, they are creating movement in Foucaultian terms, which is to say, this amalgam of resistive discourses recognizes the work of power and control that dominant blocs exert in policing the body's possibilities (Foucault, 1982), and they are actively attempting to alter the field of limitations that dictate breastfeeding.

TALKING BACK: INTERNET ACTIVISM AS FORMS OF RESISTANCE AND AS RHETORICAL TEXTS

Morrissey and Kimball (2017) provide an excellent example of how "internet technologies and social media can be used for activism and, as such, are productive sites for rhetorical inquiry" (p. 51). Morrissey and Kimball (2017) use the group "Blacktavists" to demonstrate how "shared image macros, blog posts, open letters, Facebook and status updates and Twitter hashtags" (p. 49) culminate in creating virtual activism. In a similar vein to Morrissey and Kimball (2017), our review of online resistance groups reveals a persuasive narrative that condemns friend-enemy politics of motherhood—or the mommy wars—while highlighting the numerous other kinds of motherhood existing outside of white, hegemonic femininity and the safe, healthy children those types of mothering produce. Also in line with Morrissey and Kimball (2017), we find that this "synthesis of complex cultural statements and arguments about" hegemonic mothering "into highly condensed images, phrases, and hashtags" allows groups to "spread their message quickly and widely" (p. 52). Given the control of discursive formations, these resistive pieces of rhetoric serve to upend the rules, and break the limitations, imposed by exclusive breastfeeding narratives.

"Tracing social media as a text for analysis is challenging and requires attention to not only what is being said and by whom but who is sharing, 'liking,' and reposting these cultural messages. In particular, for online messages to have resonance they must be portable, accessible, and clear" (Morrissey & Kimball, 2017, p. 52). If online collaboration is successful (liking, sharing, commenting, etc.), marginalized groups maintain a reasonable amount of control over their messages, when in other instances, like formal chains of communication, they might be overlooked and marginalized (Morrissey & Kimball, 2017).

From a critic's standpoint, the discourses of online resistance groups are "fragmented, overlapping, and complex" (Morrissey & Kimball, 2017, p. 53). To create a manageable "text," for this chapter, we gathered material from popular online personalities, groups, and bloggers and then gathered information from their shares, follows, and other collaborative online activities to identify other "resistors."

Given the interactivity between each resistor, we can argue that these fragmented texts represent social movement in light of McGee's (1983) articulation of social movement as a verb. There is a movement *away* from dialectical constructions of motherhood in these texts. There is a consensus to be inclusive rather than exclusive, to try and find comfort and confidence in one's parenting style, to accept imperfection (a concept already associated with gendered discourses) and movement *toward* collectivity. Words like "tribe" and "squad" pepper the comments sections and are often found in the image macros, articles, and videos, as well. There is also a tenor of "talking back" in hooks's (2015) terms, as a means of speaking truth to authority—to justifying one's place as an equal in a power structure that views them as subservient, or deviant. For our purposes, talking back is important, because as we alluded to in chapter 6, women who fail to embrace hegemonic femininity are not "good girls." In one sense, they have to prove they are "good enough," and at the same time, demonstrate how the rules that determine good and bad are arbitrary (or really, just patriarchal and condescending). All this suggests a collective effort to change social discourses surrounding motherhood. In this sense, pro-inclusivity mommy bloggers are reflective of Larana, Johnson, and Gusfield's (1994) definition of New Social Movements as fluid, or movements that "imply changes in how values and realities are conceived" (p. 64). Social movement from this perspective is not the organized marches or boycotts we so often think of, but rather, the everyday actions of life, which may have little to no massive public visibility (Larana, Johnson, & Gusfield, 1994). The idea of everyday action ties these social movements to a Foucaultian perspective, particularly as they relate to the technologies of the self that:

> Permit individuals to effect by their own means or with the help of others, a certain number of operations on their own bodies and souls, thoughts, conduct, and way of being, so as to transform themselves in order to attain a state of happiness, purity, wisdom, perfection or immortality. (Foucault, 1982, para. 9)

The following sections explore this vibrant, irreverent, and in our opinion, humorous group of resistors for this very purpose. We are interested in exploring how these "mommy bloggers" and online activists employ technologies of the self through virtual communication to resist discursive formations of breastfeeding so that they may transform themselves—and hopefully by extension—others into a happier, more complete, version of the self. Before doing so, we turn to an established form of media—television—to illustrate how even more traditional formats are showcasing voices of resistance.

Adam Ruins Everything

TrueTV, an American television show produced by Turner Broadcasting System, runs the popular television series, *Adam Ruins Everything.* Hosted by "investigative comedian Adam Conover," the show's website is billed as an adventure where:

> Conover embarks on a comically inventive yet unrelentingly serious quest to reveal the hidden truths behind everything you know and love. Tackling topics ranging from the workplace and voting to forensic science and security, he gives you not just fun facts to share with your friends, but information that will make you see the world in a whole new way. If knowledge is power, then Adam Conover will have you laughing all the way to the top. (*Adam Ruins Everything,* About)

We struggled with placing *Adam Ruins Everything* at the beginning of our analysis of resistance rhetorics, in part because he is a man, and while the voices of men do matter in this conversation, as feminists, we recognize the privileged place of being "first" in any analysis. As academics, we realize that most feminist and women's discourses are placed at the back of theory books. But, we are giving *Adam* a privileged place here due to an episode that aired on the topic of breastfeeding that nicely frames the reality of new mothers. This text sets a tone for the chapter from which the other resistive texts draw. The following is a description of *Adam's* episode 31, *"Why Baby Formula Isn't Poison."*

Episode 31 opens with Conover seated at a picnic table next to a young mother. Beside her is a newborn baby, nestled snugly in its car seat. Ostensibly, the scene is depicting a baby shower. The baby begins to cry, prompting the mother (Emily) to grab a bottle from a diaper bag. As she goes to remove the cap, the shot switches to the opposite side of the table where two other women sit, horrified at the sight of a mother preparing to feed her child. The first woman remarks, aghast, "Ah, wait. Is that formula?" Incredulous, the woman demands of Emily: "Tell me you're breastfeeding." It is not a question. Emily tells the women that she tried to breastfeed her baby, but explains all of the reasons it didn't work out (many of which the mothers in this book discuss). As Emily finishes, the woman across from her grabs the bottle from her hand and self-righteously announces, "Um, formula is *toxic.* You *have* to breastfeed." At this point, the other woman across from Emily chimes in, "Uh. No. I hate it when people breastfeed in public. Do that at home. Nobody wants to see that." The scene devolves into chaos as both Emily and Adam try to determine which of these two women is right, since obviously Emily—the baby's mother—is not and cannot be "right" in this discourse.

Suddenly a woman's voice shouts, "That's it!" The imposing form of Patti Murphy enters the scene! She points to the anti-breastfeeding mom. "You're gonna tell a mom where and when she can feed her baby? Get a life! Breastfeeding is normal, natural and safe." The first judgmental mother (pro-breastfeeding) raises her hand in triumph. "Preach, sister," she says smugly. Mrs. Murphy turns her attention to this mother. "And you. How dare you judge how a mom feeds her kid?" she admonishes. "Formula isn't just healthy and safe," she explains. "It's a literal life saver." Mrs. Murphy takes Emily to a child's play house, situated near the picnic table. When she opens the play house door, a sepia video of an industrial era, immigrant mother appears in the doorway. She's breastfeeding. With the image of the mother playing in the background, Mrs. Murphy explains the history of breastfeeding, the choices mothers had to make if they had issues with breastfeeding, and the number of hours a mother spent per day breastfeeding: 35 hours per week (the video uses research from Courtney Jung's 2015 work, *Lactivism*). "This is a real thing people did. Babies grew up malnourished or died if their mothers couldn't breastfeed." Mrs. Murphy then explains how the development of formula in 1865 changed the course of history for many mothers and babies. Emily looks hopeful, but then asks, Mrs. Murphy, "'Kay, but isn't formula just a bunch of chemicals?" Mrs. Murphy retorts, "Well yeah, Emily it is, because literally *everything* is a bunch of chemicals. Breast milk is also chemicals. The question is, is whether those chemicals are nutritionally different than breast milk. And the answer is no."

The viewers are introduced to Courtney Jung, the author of *Lactivist.* Jung explains all the things breast milk is supposed to aid and/or prevent: IQ, asthma, eczema, etc. "Once you account for income and education, there's almost no difference between breast feeding and formula feeding. The evidence that breastfeeding makes a difference is just inconclusive. The fact is, formula feeding is a completely safe and nutritious alternative to breastfeeding."

Episode 31 also addresses issues raised in the Nestle formula scandal by tackling the issue of safe drinking water. Mrs. Murphy explains to viewers that using clean water and sterilizing bottles is necessary for safe formula feeding. The pro-breastfeeding mother interrupts. "I read mommy blogs, like for fun, and they say that breastfeeding actually makes your baby *love* you more because it releases a bonding chemical called oxytocin." Adam responds, "Oxytocin is a hormone that gets released when you do things like hug or cuddle . . . but that same hormone is released when you do things like fire a gun or watch porn. According to a comprehensive review from 2008, there is no convincing support for a connection between breastfeeding and the quality of the mother infant relationship." Mrs. Murphy returns to the screen to say, "Breastfeeding is a great way to bond with your baby. But it's not the only one." Mrs. Murphy talks about the mothers that can't breastfeed and those that adopt. She finishes by addressing Emily, "So, the next time someone tries to guilt trip you or any other parent about how they feed their baby, you tell them they can eat my feet."

Episode 31 of *Adam Ruins Everything* exemplifies our argument throughout the book. Breastfeeding's dialectical discourses are fueled by discursive formations created through scientific and cultural discourses. But they are supported by statistics. Unfortunately, very few people truly understand statistical significance and the role of rigorous scientific design, and in the case of breast milk over formula, the research simply doesn't support the impassioned insistence some women, online bloggers, organizations, and some governmental policies promulgate. In turning from televised media to online media, we see how resistance bloggers work in tandem to "interrupt" the common sense realities created through these interwoven, exclusive breastfeeding discourses.

Moms Against Mom Shaming

Sometimes Kids Are Dicks: Online Blog.

Started by a woman named Sarah, who identifies as an "accidental mom-blogger, married to my high school sweetheart, mother to three beautiful crazy boys, frequent thrower of f-bomb," *Sometimes Kids Are Dicks,* "Is a blog about the craziness that is parenthood. The ups and downs of raising our children while maintaining our own sanity! Please join me." Sarah's blog is dedicated to highlighting the amazing highs of motherhood, and laughing at the ridiculous realities no adult expects to find themselves in. The blog is also dedicated to celebrating motherhood in all its forms and admonishes mom-shaming.

The *Sometimes Kids Are Dicks* blog is an example of McGee's (1983) notion of social movement melding with theories of online activism. At times, other "mommy bloggers" contribute to the Instagram and Facebook account, primarily by liking and sharing image macros. The postings reveal how *Sometimes Kids Are Dicks* engages with other online activism by advancing the idea that parenting should be a supportive enterprise, rather than a competition. They also reveal how infant feeding is just one aspect of parenting. Good parenting requires so much more. For example, in a July 2018 Instragram post, sometimeskidsaredicks reassures followers by reminding them that "none of our kids listen, we're all annoyed a lot, we all get angry more than we think we should. . . We all wonder if it's *THIS* hard for anyone else [but] don't for a SECOND think you're not a damn good parent. You are. Yes, I mean you." Another Instragram post from August 2018 starts with a statement, "how much I love unsolicited parenting advice," which is followed by a pie graph equally split in half between "Not at all" and "Not at all, but in red."

As these examples suggest, *Sometimes Kids Are Dicks* is committed to celebrating parenting's far from idyllic realities. It's hard. And no one is doing it perfectly. Followers are allowed to forgive themselves for their imperfections, in part, because they realize they are not alone. The memes and posts also represent a form of talking back wherein the person posting is clearly responding to a larger societal discourse—most notably discourses that are telling moms how to parent and feeling entitled to punish/judge them when they deviate from the ideals of total motherhood. This form of surveillance and disciplining by other mothers is another form of hegemonic mothering, wherein women act as their own police force. The resistors talk back to this in-group policing by demonstrating their success as parents and outing the ridiculous—and unattainable—standards of parenting hegemonic mothering adheres to. "Trying to sort out society's toxic bullshit" and "in a world where you can be anything, don't be a judgmental mom shaming twat" are just two examples which demonstrate the author's desire to be both supportive to her sisters while also calling out those who stand in judgment.

They are not the only parents imagining a sort of parenting police force handing out constant judgment. While *Sometimes Kids Are Dicks* focuses primarily on inclusivity among mothers and parenting styles, the account interacts with other accounts, like *Scary Mommy,* that specifically address breastfeeding.

Scary Mommy: Blog and Website.

> We are the history makers and the memory keepers.
> We are the snot catchers and the ass wipers.
> We've seen it all, heard it all, and smelled it all,
> but we wouldn't have it any other way.
> We are millions of unique women, united by motherhood.
> We are scary, and we are proud. (Scary Mommy, About, 2017)

These lines grace *Scary Mommy's* homepage. They are the first writings visitors see when they visit the page. Proud and unapologetic are just two words that resonate throughout the articles, websites, and social media pages that make up the *Scary Mommy* enterprise. The organization's Instagram page is full of empowering messages, sometimes shared from other mommy bloggers, like *Sometimes Kids Are Dicks,* or *Mommy Cusses,* and is supported by online articles that help mothers recognize their potential despite their imperfections. For instance, in one of her Instagram posts she asserts, "When I see a mom who's barely holding her shit together by a thread, I know I've found my people" (*Scary Mommy,* February 21, 2018, [Instagram post]).

According to the website's history, "*Scary Mommy*" was started by Jill Smokler in early 2008 as an "innocent online baby book to chronicle her stay-at-home days with her children. It transformed into a massive vibrant community of millions of parents, brought together by a common theme: Parenting doesn't have to be perfect" (Scary Mommy, About). Scary Mommy was acquired by Some Spider media company in 2015 (Scary Mommy, About). In that time, Smokler and other writers for the company have dedicated their time to "creating and curating online content for parents, having grown her one-time 'mommy blog' into one of the most influential digital parenting properties in the world" (Scary Mommy, About). The content they produce is both funny and heart wrenching, "compelling and sometimes controversial," which resulted in "a new kind of digital parenting ecosystem that has given moms a voice and brands a roadmap for engaging the sought after mom audience" (Smokler, N/D).

Scary Mommy's success and influence is impactful because so many other mothers and parents follow the posts, blogs, and articles for guidance and support. And they derive emotional sustenance from these forms of communication. They gain confidence in their own lived experiences and are able to see their performance of parenting as existing within the boundaries of acceptable parenting. When it comes to breastfeeding, *Scary Mommy* is supportive of choice, not exclusivity. In a February 2017 article, "Mom's Honest Post Speaks to Every Mother Whose Struggled with Breastfeeding," Sarah Hosseini writes about a mother who went viral with her breastfeeding struggles and the fallout she endured: "We all so desperately want to survive and push through. We so badly want to have our baby thrive. We want that relationship," she writes. "We want the experience. In the end, fed is best. That's what matters" (Hosseini, 2017). Hosseini concludes, "That's the truth bomb right there: all moms want what is best for their babies. Getting them fed—no matter how—is the universal and ultimate goal for parents" (para. 8).

Another article speaks to the overwhelming pressure mothers feel to be perfect. The article's author, Ilyse Dobrow DiMarco (N/D), writes:

> The common thread that weaves my story together with those I mentioned above—maternal feelings of inadequacy and guilt. In CBT, we talk about people "should"-ing all over themselves, bombarding them-

> selves with self-talk about all the things they should be doing and aren't. "Should"-ing leads directly to guilt and shame. And many moms are consumed with "shoulds" about breastfeeding, and the shame and guilt that come with them, whether they ultimately decide to nurse or not. (para. 10)

DiMarco's story leads to an important narrative that is consistent among resistant breastfeeding narratives: Self-reflection/actualization through experience.

> I ultimately had to recognize that it was unfair to compare myself to her. I absolutely respected this woman's decision to keep nursing, but I knew that our values were different. I believed in nursing, but I could not identify with someone who felt so strongly about nursing that she sacrificed her own health and well-being for the cause. I also recognized that I did not know this woman and therefore could not pass judgment on her choice to nurse through the pain. In other words, my experience was totally different than hers. I couldn't compare myself to her. (DiMarco, N/D, para. 11)

DiMarco's narrative embraces a feminist ethic of experiential knowledge and reinforces a dynamic, multivocal narrative of the feminine experience rather than setting limits through strict discursive formations.

Lisa Sadikman (N/D) embraces the idea of mother-centered versus baby-friendly rhetoric in her reflections on breastfeeding:

> So don't ask about breastfeeding.
>
> If you're truly concerned about how life is going with a baby in the mix, there's adifferent question you can ask: *How are you doing?* (para. 7–9)

> What moms really need is to feel cared for and supported. What they need is a support system. They need the love and understanding of family and friends, doctors, neighbors, strangers and yes, even the guy behind the deli counter. In those delicate first days, weeks and months of motherhood, women need to know they will not be judged or criticized for the way they feel or how they choose to mother their babies. However, a mama feeds her baby is the right way. Making her feel otherwise is unkind and counterproductive. (para. 10)

Christine Organ's (N/D) article, "Breastfeeding is Wonderful, but Mom's Health and Happiness Matter, Too" also encourages more mother-centric narratives. Her article begins with the statistical benefits of breastfeeding, but continues with:

> These statistics are just that—statistics. And numbers can never tell the whole story. Numbers don't show the pain—like shards of glass through your nipples—that some women feel when they breastfeed. Statistics don't show the tears shed when a mother struggles with low-supply or latching problems. And data can't measure the shame a

> mother is often overcome with if she chooses not to (or can't) breastfeed. (para. 1)

Organ continues by addressing the recommendations for breastfeeding as determined by international breastfeeding organizations, The American Academy of Pediatrics, and The American Academy of Obstetricians. She is careful to note that recommendations are not edicts:

> But these recommendations fail to address the individual needs of a mother, baby, and family. They don't consider the emotional and physical challenges—not to mention the long-term scars that can remain if breastfeeding doesn't work out for any number of reasons. They make no mention of the vitally important mother-baby bond that requires first and foremost a secure, stable, happy mom. (para. 5)

She notes that some doctors, who are also mothers, "blame the health care system for 'collud[ing] to ignore the individual circumstances of mothers in order to promote a one-size fits all prescription: breast milk-only nutrition for infants,'" (para. 12) and notes

> Breastfeeding is about more than nutrition , after all; it's also about cuddling and feeling emotionally connected to the baby so that the child feels safe, comfortable, and connected to the surrounding world. This can be accomplished, the doctors say, in a number of ways. The guidelines are based on legitimate science, of course, but they also carry a threat (if you don't breastfeed, your baby is at risk) and a stigma (if you don't breastfeed, you're not a good mother), both of which can be detrimental for many mothers. (para. 13)

Quoting the mother/doctors who contributed to her article, Organ tells readers, "Just as new babies are vulnerable, so are their mothers," (as cited in Organ, N/D, para. 14). "And a mother's mental health is crucial—not just to her, but also to her baby. A depressed and anxious mother isn't able to provide the nurturing that her baby needs to develop and grow" (para. 14).

Contributors to Scary Mommy also address the heuristic of the natural. For example, Scagell (2018) writes about the fall-out from *Target*'s decision to label the breastfeeding supplies aisle as the "Natural Feeding" section of the store. For some, reacting online through social media posting, *Target's* labeling was consistent and accurate: breastfeeding is natural. It should be labeled as such. For others, because of the association with all things natural being "better," labeling the aisle as "natural" reinforced a dialectic that situated formula feeding as a less desirable or defective method of infant care. The online debate was intense, and as demonstrated by Scagell's (2018) research, reified claims that mothers police each other. Scagell (2018) addresses the mommy war mentality brewing online with the following:

> though it appears this is only how Target labels this section in their stores and not online, it obviously struck a chord with many. Regardless of how we feed our children, all moms seem to face some sort of criticism about this intensely personal decision. Moms who breastfeed are continuously called out in public and told to cover up and those who decide to bottle-feed are often ridiculed and told they aren't doing what's best for their child. (para. 6)

Scagell (2018) concludes the piece with the following:

> I think a better use of everyone's time is to be asking one another how best we can support each other in *every* aspect of motherhood, feeding included. It's not an easy journey and having love without judgment can sometimes make all the difference. Only you know what's best for you and your child, end of story. We need more ways to draw people together, not tear each other down. (para. 7)

Just as bottle feeding doesn't equal failure, *Scary Mommy* contributors are quick to point out that breastfeeding doesn't equal success. In her article, "Breastfeeding does not equal success in Motherhood," Tiffany Wright discusses feeling shame while buying formula. She talks about furtively walking the aisle, hoping no one would see her or realize what she was doing. Then it hit her. She shouldn't feel *any* way. Her baby was hungry and needed to eat. She was taking care of that issue (Wright, N/D). But her options—and feelings—were limited and policed by the discursive formations that formed her realities of motherhood:

> *Why do I feel so much shame for giving my baby a bottle?* I believe there are more than a few contributing factors. In the circles I grew up in, breastfeeding was it. I knew moms who exclusively nursed their babies until they were 2 or 3 years old. While I support mothers in their right to choose, there seemed to be an unspoken judgment on anyone who didn't follow their example. "So how long do you plan on breastfeeding?" they ask, as if bottle feeding hasn't crossed their mind a day in their life. When I lost my milk supply back in April, the few people who knew about it pushed me to do every possible thing to bring it back. While I appreciated their encouragement in my decision to breastfeed from day one, it became a little less like support and a little more like pressure. (Wright, N/D, para. 10–11)

Wright goes on to talk about leaving breastfeeding Facebook groups, because even though they were unaware she was no longer breastfeeding, she knew she was the bad mother they were all talking about:

> We have a few precious pictures of my husband feeding our son that I never posted only because of the condemnation I worried people would cast upon us. Looking back, I realize all of this was absolutely ridiculous. Yes, breastfeeding does have many benefits, both emotional and physical. But if I'm so focused on trying to force it that it takes

> away the beauty of what I'm doing (nourishing a baby human) then I need to stop. (para. 15)

Wright needed to stop trying to exclusively breastfeed, she says, because she was losing quality time with her baby while she tried to meet a standard of perfection that is 1) unreasonable; and 2) unnecessary. She realized that this time with her infant will all too quickly slip away:

> Bottle-feeding will not cause my baby to struggle with bonding. It will not make my baby sick, nor make him feel loved any less. If his belly is full, I am a good mother. Repeat that out loud. If his belly is full, I am a good mother. (para. 16)

Wright lost her milk supply naturally but she tells mothers that no matter why they are bottle feeding, they are not bad mothers. Perhaps in response to the Facebook moms who couldn't accept her form of mothering, Wright finishes her article by stating, "Breastfeeding does not always equal success in motherhood" (Wright, para. 18). This statement introduces a moment of interruption for us. There is so much more to motherhood than infant feeding. Breastfeeding narratives have policed motherhood so completely that we very rarely talk about all the other things that make us great mothers and parents.

In the spirit of embracing those "other" parenting qualities, *Scary Mommy* articles sometimes introduce new studies in child and infant care that help readers shift the focus from breastfeeding. In one article, contributors challenge the Breast-is-Best narrative with new data suggesting breastfeeding benefits wane by age 5, and aren't necessarily providing long-term cognitive development.

> Again—it wasn't *better*. And why are we so stuck on what's *better*, anyway? Wouldn't it be fantastic if we could once and for all drop the "Breast is Best" mantra, so all women could be made to feel confident about their choices, rather than shamed for not making the "best" one? Wouldn't it be great if there didn't need to be a "better" choice? (Guido, para. 5)

The article's author goes on to discuss other factors that increase infant well-being, including a mother's wealth, health, and education level. Much like the *Adam Ruins Everything* episode, this article examines motherhood with a holistic approach, not a breast-centric approach.

Sometimes, *Scary Mommy* stories rely on pathos to help mothers understand the complexity of motherhood in an effort to guide women toward more civilized conversations. For example, Sara Lindborg, shares her gut-wrenching story with readers in a manner that invokes sympathy and understanding, rather than judgement and admonishment:

> My daughter was not gaining, in fact, she was losing—fast. We agreed to try a SNS (a tube system that fed her formula while she nursed). We fed our daughter with a syringe, so as not to have nipple confusion. I

> took away her pacifier so she would crave my nipples more. I pumped my breasts until they were bruised in order to produce an ounce for her. Just the smallest amount to give her the nutrition I thought she needed; the only nutrition that I would allow myself to give her. (para. 4)
>
> We spent hours hooked up to a machine, researching herbs, buying medicine that can only be purchased in other countries. (para. 5)
>
> Looking back at it now, I sacrificed her health for my pride. I would not give up. I would not supplement with formula. She was hungry and I was torn. I can still remember the first night we gave her formula from a bottle: I cried and she slept. (para. 6)

Speaking about her second child, Lindborg again describes how hard she tried to breastfeed, and how awful it felt. In retrospect she reveals:

> My son just turned 6-years-old and it has taken that long to open up about this, to let go of the feelings of disappointment, failure, guilt, embarrassment and inadequacy, to recognize that I was angry and hurt that I could not produce enough milk to feed my babies. (para. 13)
>
> What I have come to realize is that I failed my children, not because I couldn't exclusively nurse them, but because I couldn't get out of my own way. (para. 14)

She concludes:

> What I do know for sure is that all is not lost on that experience—what I have learned is invaluable. Women must trust their instincts and believe in what their body is telling them. Consider what others say, but ultimately do what feels right. (para. 15)

In conversation with the *Adam Ruins Everything* episode, Annie Reneau, our final *Scary Mommy* contributor, describes herself as "Big-honking-breastfeeding fan," (Reneau, N/D para. 1) but asks breastfeeding advocates to cease the following:

- Arguing with moms who say they were unable to breastfeed.
- Acting like formula is poison.
- Assuming that someone who didn't breastfeed doesn't know the facts.
- Refusing to sympathize with people who are uncomfortable with breastfeeding.
- Letting your passion about breastfeeding come out as snark.

Meghan Koziel's story is just one of the reasons we agree with Reneau and her tips for breastfeeding advocates. Koziel's story is one of sacrifice and survival. It is also an example of resistance to breastfeeding that embodies a feminist ethic of subversion through experience.

Koziel was diagnosed with breast cancer at the age of 26. She lost both breasts in her struggle to beat the disease, which she ultimately did do.

Two years later, Koziel and her husband announced the impending birth of their first child. Knowing the scrutiny she would face, Koziel created the following banner and hung it over her hospital bed (see Figure 7.1).

According to McLain (2018), Koziel explained the banner as a means to support other survivors and to stave off hospital staff eager to promote Baby-Friendly policies:

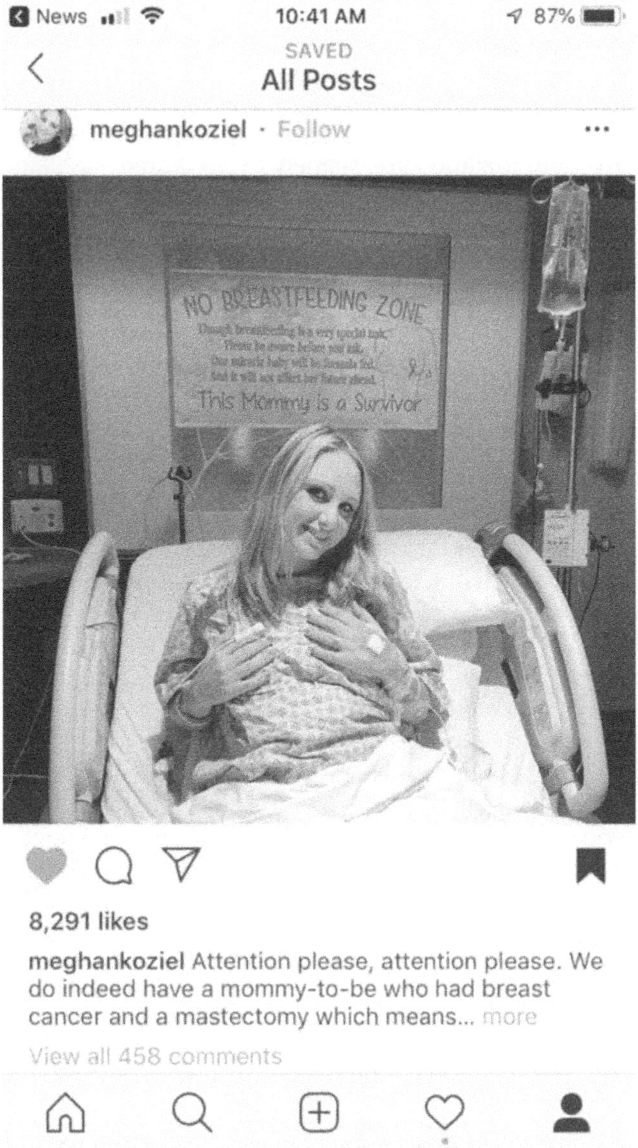

Figure 7.1. Meghan Koziel, September 14, 2018 [Instagram photo]. Retrieved from https://www.instagram.com/p/BnumLoeBWtA/?utm_source=ig_embed_).

> I got the idea to make a banner from one of my followers who also had a baby post-mastectomy and felt "formula shamed" by hospital staff. It would be heartbreaking enough to have my baby reflexively rooting for my breast when I am physically incapable of breastfeeding her. I didn't want anyone pushing their breastfeeding views onto me without knowing my history. So I wanted to come up with something subtle to let them know, but also direct enough to get my point across. (as cited in McLain, 2018)

Taking Back the Meaning of Motherhood

We are not knowledgeable simply by the reality of our birth (Hall, 1997). Rather, our realities are shaped by a shared language (see the Sapir-Whorf hypothesis), or a conceptual map (Hall, 1997). Foucault reminds us that we become knowledgeable (cultured) by learning the systems and codes of our language/culture (Gordon, 1980). As members of a particular culture, we each have a conceptual map that we use to guide us through discursive situations. When our maps are similar, we can make sense of each other and the values, morals, and beliefs that we hold. But as we've demonstrated throughout our discussions of Foucault, discursive formations, and breastfeeding, this understanding requires a common language or "linguistic relativism" (Hall, 1997).

Throughout this book, we have paid particular attention to the rules of language that limit possibilities. In this chapter, we have taken care to show the mediated performances of those trying to broaden the limitations placed on women when they feed their children. The consumer resistance movements that countered formula maker's unethical marketing practices forced wide scale—and much needed—industry change. However, while perhaps a latent effect, the resulting infant feeding discourses helped to sustain a growing hegemonic discourse of the heuristic of the natural, and further fueled the Mommy War flames. Well intended words and actions re-shaped meaning and created a new hegemonic discourse for women and their children.

Things don't mean; they are constructed (constructionist approach) and representation is the construction of meaning through language (Gordon, 1980; Hall, 1997) All meanings are produced within history and culture. It is not what is happening in front of us that matters. It's the spectacle, or the meanings and representations of social actors—both negative and positive—that is important (Hall, 1997). If successful femininity is the result of post-feminist "empowerment narratives constrained within the heterosexual matrix, norms of racial hierarchy, and normative understandings of femininity" (Favre, 2015 p. 639), then our task is to reveal the persuasiveness of these narratives. As Favre (2015) explains, "figures of hegemonic femininity need to be critically explored as sites where narratives of empowerment and constraint intersect, acting to display the boundaries of femininity in a cultural moment emphasizing choice, individualism, and success" (p. 639) as they are associated with gender, race, and class. Breastfeeding mothers are rewarded precisely because they perform within the same social hierarchies.

In the case of breastfeeding, we are constantly confronted with the spectacle (women, breasts, bottles, and babies). It is up to us to determine what that spectacle means. For the women, writers, online posters and participators, and other activists discussed in this chapter, the spectacle of the breast has taken on new meaning when it comes to motherhood, and these women want to remember that meaning in more inclusive ways. Their method of resistance is uniquely feminist in that is collective, embraces choice and change, and welcomes a cacophony of voices in the hopes of creating a more complete, diverse, and hopeful discourse of breastfeeding.

These individuals as well as those moms whose voices you "heard" in this book are starting to crack the current Breast-is-Best Discursive Formation. They are creating new discourses—ones that are less myopically focused on exclusive breastfeeding and more attentive to the multi-vocality of infant care. Our wish is that this book is one more voice, another contributor to a new discourse that begins by interrogating the hegemonic nature of the current pro-breastfeeding paradigm. It is our hope that such work will foster attempts that help mothers and their families regain their own agency when it comes to choosing how to best nourish their babies. To empower women to take back their bodies, their breasts. Armed with newer medical science that is revealing some nonsignificant differences between bottle feeding and breastfeeding, we envision a world where all parents are given the space to choose the form of nourishment that works best for them and their baby. Society can certainly help by providing information on the options available, but we would prefer that it not be so uni-vocal and oppressive in its stance. In no way are we discouraging women from breastfeeding, for we certainly embrace its benefits for baby, mom, and family. However, we do want to encourage people to afford parents the freedom of choice with regard to feeding their babies—to allow them the agency and respect to make a decision that is right for them.

References

1990–2005 Celebrating the Innocenti Declaration on the protection, promotion and support of breastfeeding: Past achievements, present challenges and the way forward for infant and young child feeding. (2005). Florence, Italy: UNICEF Innocenti Research Centre.
A structural race analysis of first food. (2015). Center for Social Inclusion: New York.
American Association of University Women. (N/D). The simple truth about the gender paygap. *Economic Security*. Retrieved from https://www.aauw.org/research/the-simple-truth-about-the-gender-pay-gap/.
American Association of University Women. (N/D). Know your rights: Title VII of the Civil Rights Act of 1964. Retrieved from https://www.aauw.org/what-we-do/legal-resources/know-your-rights-at-work/title-vii/.
Anstey, E. H., Chen, J., Elam-Evans, L. D., & Perrine, C. G. (July 14, 2017). Race and geographic differences in breastfeeding—United States, 2011–2015. Centers for Disease Control & Prevention; Morbidity and Mortality Weekly Report, 66, 723–727.
Applebome, P. (May 15, 2007). Jerry Falwell, leading religious conservative, dies. *New York Times*. Retrieved from https://www.nytimes.com/2007/05/15/obituaries/15cndfalwell.html.
Baby-friendly hospitals promoted under new project with the CDC. (October 9, 2014) Retrieved from Cision PRWeb http://www.prweb.com/releases/2014/10/prweb12237878.htm.
Baby-Friendly USA. (2010). *About the BFHI*. Retrieved on October 20, 2011 from http://www.babyfriendlyusa.org/eng/01.html.
Baby-Friendly USA. (2016). *Guidelines and Evaluation Criteria for Facilities Seeking Baby-Friendly Designation*. Albany, NY: Baby-Friendly USA.
BabyCenter.com. (July 2017). Top baby costs, and how to save. Retrieved from https://www.babycenter.com/top-baby-costs.
Baer, H. (2016). Redoing feminism: Digital activism, body politics, and neoliberalism, *Feminist Media Studies, 16*, 1, 17–34, doi: 10.1080/14680777.2015.1093070
Black, S.E., Whitmore Schanzenbach, D., & Breitwieser, A. (2017). The recent decline in women's labor force participation. *The Hamilton Project*. Retrieved from http://www.hamiltonproject.org/papers/the_recent_decline_in_womens_labor_force_participation.
Blume, L. (1999). *At the breast: Ideologies of breastfeeding and motherhood in the contemporary United States*. Boston: Beacon Press.
Bobel, C. (2001). Bounded liberation: A focused study of La Leche International. *Gender & Society, 15*, 1, 130–151. doi: 10.1177/089124301015001007
Brady, J. P. (2012). Marketing breast milk substitutes: Problems and perils throughout the world. *Archives of Disease in Childhood, 97*, 529–532.
Breastfeeding Report Card. (2014). Retrieved from https://www.cdc.gov/breastfeeding/pdf/2014breastfeedingreportcard.pdf.
Brown, L. P., Bair, A. H., & Meier, P. P. (2003). Does federal funding for breastfeeding research target our national health objectives. *Pediatrics*, 111, 4, 360–364.
Burke, A. (December 5, 2017). 10 facts about American women in the workforce. *Brookings*. Retrieved from https://www.brookings.edu/blog/brookings-now/2017/12/05/10-facts-aboutamerican-women-in-the-workforce/.
Burke, K. (1969). *A rhetoric of motives*. Berkeley, University of California Press.
Butler, J. (2004). *Undoing gender*. New York: Routledge.

Centers for Disease Control and Prevention. (August 2018). Breastfeeding Among U.S. Children Born 2009–2015, CDC National Immunization Survey. Retrieved December 17, 2018 from https://www.cdc.gov/breastfeeding/data/nis_data/results.html.

Christian Family Movement. (2009). About. Retrieved from https://www.cfm.org/about.

Cohen, S. (August 26, 2015). The day women went on strike. *Time Magazine*. Retrieved from http://time.com/4008060/women-strike-equality-1970/.

Collins, P. H. (1990). *Black feminist thought: Knowledge, consciousness and the politics of empowerment*. Boston, MA: Unwin Hyman.

Congressional Research Service Reports. (May 18, 2018). Women in Congress: Statistics and a brief overview. Retrieved from https://www.everycrsreport.com/files/20180508_R43244_27641671f850c1b441f6f543b96731949baae7f.pdf.

Conover, A. (2015–present). *Adam ruins everything*. [Television Series]. TrueTV.

Country experiences with the Baby-Friendly Hospital Initiative: Compendium of case studies from around the world. (2017). New York: UNICEF and WHO.

Crook, M. (2017). *Thicker than blood: Adoptive parenting in the modern world*. Vancouver, British Columbia: Arsenal Pulp Press.

Delli Fraine, J., Langabeer II, J., Delgado, R., Williams, J. F., & Gong, A. (2013). A transition strategy for becoming a baby-friendly hospital: Exploring the costs, benefits, and challenges. *Breastfeeding Medicine*, April 2013. Ahead of print. http://doi.org.libproxy.uncg.edu/10.1089/bfm.2012.0050.

DiMarco, D. (N/D). Stop telling moms how they 'should' be breastfeeding. *Scary Mommy*. Retrieved from https://www.scarymommy.com/breastfeeding-shoulds/.

Douglas, S., & Michaels, M. (2004). The mommy myth: The idealization of motherhood and how it has undermined women. New York: Simon & Schuster.

Dreyfus, H. L., & Rabinow, P. (1982). *Michel Foucault: Beyond structuralism and hermeneutics*. Chicago: The University of Chicago Press.

Edwards P. N. (2004). Why can't women just say no? And does it really matter? In M. Kirkham (Ed.), *Informed choice in maternity care* (pp. 1–22). New York: Palgrave Macmillan.

Ember, C., & Ember, M. (2003). *Encyclopedia of sex and gender*. Boston, MA: Springer.

Executive Order 10980 (December 14, 1961). Presidential status on the status of women.

Fairclough, N. (1989). *Language and power*. New York: Longman.

Fairclough, N. (1996). Rhetoric and critical discourse analysis: A reply to Titus Ensink and Chritsoph Saur. *Current Issues in Language and Society, 3,* 3, 286–289.

Favre, J. (2015). A maternal heart: Angelina Jolie, choices of maternity, and hegemonic femininity in *People* magazine. *Feminist and Media Studies, 15,* 4, 626–642.

Foucault, M. (1972). *The Archaeology of knowledge*. Paris: Éditions Gallimard

Foucault, M. (1979). *Discipline and punish*. New York: Vintage Books.

Foucault, M. (1982). *Technologies of the self*. [Lecture]. University of Vermont. Retrieved from https://foucault.info/documents/foucault.technologiesOfSelf.en/.

Foucault, M. (1984). The order of discourse. In M. Shapiro (Ed.), *Language and politics* (pp. 108–138). Oxford: Blackwell.

Foucault, M. (1990). *The history of sexuality. Volume 1: An introduction* (Vintage Books Ed.). New York: Vintage Books.

Foucault, M. (1994a). *The birth of the clinic: An archaeology of medical perception* (Vintage Books Ed.). New York: Vintage Books.

Foucault, M. (1994b). *The order of things: An archeology of human sciences*. New York: Knopf Doubleday Publishing Group.

Foucault, M. (1995). *Discipline and punish: The birth of the prison* (Vintage Books 2nd. Ed.). New York: Vintage Books.

Foucault, M. (2010a). *The archaeology of knowledge and the discourse of language* (Vintage Books Ed.). New York: Vintage Books.

Foucault, M. (2010b). *The order of things: An archeology of the human sciences*. New York: Vintage Books.

Foust, C. R. (2008). Aesthetics as weapons in the 'War of Ideas': Exploring the digital and typographic in American conservative web sites. *Southern Communication Journal, 73*, 2, 122–142.

Gordon, C. (Ed.) (1980). *Power/knowledge: Selecting interviews and other writings 1972–1977 Michel Foucault*. New York: Pantheon Books.

Guido, M. (March 2017). New study shows cognitive benefits of breastfeeding are negligible by age five. *Scary Mommy*, https://www.scarymommy.com/new-study-shows-cognitive-benefitsof-breastfeeding-are-negligible-by-age-five/.

Hall, S. (1997). The work of representation. In S. Hall (Ed.), *Representation: Cultural representations and signifying practices* (pp. 13–74). Thousand Oaks, CA: Sage Publications.

Hall, S. (2001). Foucault: Power, knowledge, and discourse. In M. Wetherel, S. Taylor, & S. J. Yates (Eds.), *Discourse, theory, and practice: A reader* (pp. 72–80). Thousand Oaks, CA: Sage Publications.

Hart, R. (1997). *Modern rhetorical criticism*. New York: Simon & Schuster.

Hauser, S. (May 15, 2012) The women's movement in the '70s, today: 'You've come a long way,' but . . . *Workforce*. Retrieved from https://www.workforce.com/2012/05/15/the-womens-movement-in-the-70s-today-youve-come-a-long-way-but/.

Hausman, B. (2000). Rational management: Medical authority and ideological conflict in Ruth Lawrence's breastfeeding: A guide for the medical profession. *Technical Communication Quarterly, 9*, 3, 271–289.

Hays, S. (1996). *The cultural contradictions of motherhood*. New Haven, Yale University Press.

HHS blueprint for action on breastfeeding (2000). Washington, DC: U.S. Department of Health & Human Services.

Hill Collins, P. (2007). Shifting the center: Race, class and feminist theorizing about motherhood. In A. O'Reilly (Ed.), *Maternal theory: Essential Readings* (pp. 311–330). Bradford, Canada: Demeter Press.

Hipple, S. F. (September 2016). Labor force participation: What has happened since the peak? *Monthly Labor Review*. Retrieved from https://www.bls.gov/opub/mlr/2016/article/pdf/labor-force-participation-what-has-happened-since-the-peak.pdf.

Hirschman C., & Butler, M. (1981). Trends and differentials on breastfeeding: An update. *Demography, 18*, 1, 39–54.

History, Art, and Archives: United States House of Representatives. The Year of the Woman. 1992. Retrieved from http://history.house.gov/Exhibitions-and-Publications/WIC/Historical-Essays/Assembling-Amplifying-Ascending/Women-Decade/.

hooks, b. (2015). *Talking back: Thinking feminist, thinking black*. Routledge: New York.

Hosseini, S. (February 2, 2017). Mom's Honest Post Speaks to Every Mother Who's Struggled With Breastfeeding. *Scary Mommy*. Retrieved from https://www.scarymommy.com/moms-honest-breastfeeding-post/.

Howorth, C. (October 19, 2017). Motherhood is hard to get wrong. So why do so many moms feel so bad about themselves? *Time Magazine*. Retrieved from https://time.com/magazine/us/4989032/october-30th-207-vol-190-no-18-u-s/.

Hulbert, A. (2003). *Raising America: Experts, parents, and a century of advice about children*. New York: Alfred A. Knopf.

Human Rights Watch. (June 20, 2017). US: New York Governor signs anti-child marriage law. Retrieved from https://www.hrw.org/news/2017/06/20/us-new-york-governor-signs-anti-child-marriage-law.

Innocenti declaration on the protection, promotion, and support of breastfeeding. (1990). New York City: UNICEF.

International code of marketing of breast-tmilk substitutes. (1981). Geneva, Switzerland: World Health Organization.

Jones, K. M., Power, M. L., Queenan, J. T., & Schulkin, J. (2015). Racial and ethnic disparities in breastfeeding. *Breastfeeding Medicine*, 14, 186–196. doi: 10.1089/bfm.2014.0152

Jung, C. (2015). *Lactivism: How feminists and fundamentalists, hippies and yuppies, and physicians and politicians made breastfeeding big business and bad policy*. New York: Basic Books.

Karlgaard, R. (March 11, 2010). *The not so great recession*. Retrieved July 12, 2018 from https://www.forbes.com/forbes/2010/0329/opinions-rich-karlgaard-great-recession-digital-rules.html#4a623c3e50b7.

Koerber, A. (2006). Rhetorical agency, resistance, and the disciplinary rhetorics of breastfeeding. *Technical Communication Quarterly, 15*, 87–101.

Kotler, A. (2006). Ethics of distributing commercial gift bags to new mothers. *American Academy of Pediatrics*. Retrieved March 22, 2007 from www.aap.org.

Koziel, M. (September 14, 2018) [Instagram photo] https://www.instagram.com/p/BnumLoeBWtA/?utm_source=ig_embed_).

Kramer, M. S., Fombonne, E., Igumnov, S., Vanilovich, I., Matush, L., Mironova, E., Bogdanovich, N., Tremblay, R. E., Chalmers, B., Zhang, X., & Platt, R. W. (2008). Effects of prolonged and exclusive breastfeeding on child behavior and maternal adjustment: Evidence from a large, randomized trial. *Pediatrics, 121*, e435–e440.

Krasny, J. (June 25, 2012). Every parent should know the scandalous history of infant formula. Retrieved from https://www.businessinsider.com/nestles-infant-formula-scandal-2012-6.

Ladd-Taylor, M., & Umansky, L. (1998). *BAD MOTHERS: The politics of blame in twentieth century America*. New York: NYU Press.

Larana, E., Johnson, H., & Gusfield, J. R. (1994). New social movements: From ideology to identity. Philadelphia, PA: Temple University Press.

Largo Janssen, T. (2007). Sex, gender and health: Developments in research. *European Journal of Women's Studies, 14*, 1, 9–20.

La Leche League International, "History." Retrieved June 22, 2018 from https://www.llli.org/about/history/.

La Leche League International. (2011a). A brief history of La Leche League International. Retrieved from https://www.llli.org/about/history/.

La Leche League International. (2011b). Chapter one. In *The womanly Art of Breastfeeding*. Penguin Random House Canada. Retrieved from https://www.penguinrandomhouse.ca/books/196502/the-womanly-art-of-breastfeeding-by-la-leche-league-international/9780345518446/excerpt.

La Leche League International. Philosophy. Retrieved from https://www.llli.org/about/philosophy/.

MacDonald, T., Noel-Weiss, J., West, D., Walks, M., Biener, M., Kibbe A., & Myler, E. (2016). Transmasculine individuals' experiences with lactation, chestfeeding, and gender identity: A qualitative study. *BMC Pregnancy and Childbirth, 16*, 106 doi: 10.1186/s12884-016-0907-y

McAllister, J. (2017). The complete guide to everything you need to know about a healthy pregnancy that fits your lifestyle and heals your body after childbirth. Amazon Digital Services.

McGee, M. (1983). Social movement as meaning. *Central States Speech Journal, 34*, 1, 74–77.

McGee, M. C. (1980). 'Social movement': Phenomenon or meaning? In C. E. Morris & S. H. Brown, *Readings on the rhetoric of protest* (pp. 125–136). State College, PA: Strata Publishing, State College.

McGeough, A., & Rudick, K. C. (2018). 'It was at the library; therefore it must be credible': Mapping patterns of undergraduate heuristic decision-making. *Education*, 67, 2, 165–184.

McLain, A. (October 22, 2018). This cancer survivor put a 'No Breastfeeding Zone' in her delivery room and here's why. *Buzzfeed*. Retrieved from https://www.buzzfeed.com/asiawmclain/cancer-survivor-no-breastfeeding-banner.

McLaren, M. A. (2002). *Feminism, Foucault and embodied subjectivity*. New York: State University of New York Press.

McRobbie, A. (2004). Post-feminism and popular culture. *Feminist Media Studies, 4,* 255–264.
McRobbie, A. (2009). *The aftermath of feminism: Gender, culture and social change.* Thousand Oaks, CA: Sage Publications.
McVicar, M. (2016). The religious right in America. *Oxford Research Encyclopedia of Religion.* Ed. Retrieved November 1, 2018, from http://religion.oxfordre.com/view/10.1093/acrefore/9780199340378.001.0001/acrefore-9780199340378-e-97.
Morrissey, M. E., & Kimball, K. Y. (2017). #SpoiledMilk: Blacktavists, visibility, and the exploitation of the black breast. *Women's Studies in Communication, 40,* 48–66, doi: 10.1080/07491409.2015.1121945
Murkoff, H., & Mazel, S. (2014). *What to expect in the first year.* New York: Workman Publishing.
Murkoff, H., & Mazel, S. (2016). *What to expect when you're expecting.* New York: Workman Publishing.
Muscato, Annie Ferguson. (April 16, 2016). In *Facebook.* Retrieved December 20, 2018, from https://www.facebook.com/annie.cferguson/posts/10206014803904620.
Nadesan, M. H., & Sotirin, P. (1998). The romance and science of "Breast is Best": Discursive contradictions and contexts of breast-feeding choices. *Text & Performance Quarterly, 18,* 217–232.
National Broadcast Association Nightly News. (October 29, 1984). The rise of the religious right. [video]. Retrieved from https://highered.nbclearn.com/portal/site/HigherEd/flatview?cuecard=5143.
National Family Planning and Reproductive Health Association. Domestic gag rule: Challenges for Title X patients and providers. Retrieved from https://www.nationalfamilyplanning.org/file/Domestic-Gag-Fact-Sheet.pdf.
Niewert, D. (2017). *Alt-America: The rise of the radical right in the age of Trump.* Verso.
Northrup, C. (2010). *Women's bodies, women's wisdom: Creating physical and emotional health and healing.* New York: Bantam Books.
Norton, A. J., & Miller, L. F. (1992). *Marriage, divorce, and remarriage in the 1990's. Current Population Reports, Population Characteristics, 180,* i-1–21. U.S. National Library of Medicine. National Institutes of Health. Retrieved from https://www.ncbi.nlm.nih.gov/pubmed/12345021.
Organ, C. (N/D). Breastfeeding is wonderful, but Mom's health and happiness matter, too. *Scary Mommy.* Retrieved from https://www.scarymommy.com/breastfeeding-affects-moms-health-happiness/.
Our Bodies, Our Choices Blogspot. (2012). http://obocnow.blogspot.com/2012/04/timeline-of-reproductive-rights.html.
Pederson, C., & Effron, L. (2012). 'What to expect when you're expecting': Top 10 changes in the new edition." *ABC News: Nightline.* Retrieved from https://abcnews.go.com/Health/expect-expecting-top-10-edition/story?id=16320518.
Perelman, C., & Olbrechts-Tyteca, L. (1969). *The new rhetoric: A treatise on argumentation.* Notre Dame: University of Notre Dame Press.
Phillips, N., & Hardy, C. (2002). *Discourse analysis: Investigating processes of social construction.* Thousand Oaks, CA: Sage.
Quart, A. (2012). *The milk wars.* Retrieved from https://www.nytimes.com/2012/07/15/opinion/sunday/the-breast-feeding-wars.html?_r=3&partner=rss&emc=rssI.
Rabinow, P. (1984). Introduction. In P. Rabinow (Ed.), The Foucault reader (pp. 3–29). New York: Pantheon Books.
Radford, G. P. (2003). Trapped in our own discursive formations: Toward an archaeology of library and information science. *The Library Quarterly, 73,* 1–18.
Reneau, A. (N/D). 5 things breastfeeding advocates should never do. *Scary Mommy.com.* Retrieved from https://www.scarymommy.com/breastfeeding-advocates-should-never/.
Rippey, P. L. F., & Falconi, L. (2017). A land of milk and honey? Breastfeeding and identity in lesbian families. *Journal of GLBT Family Studies, 13,* 16–39.

Rodgers, O. (2015). 'Relinquish the reins': Persuasion and consensus in the discourse of pregnancy and childbirth advice literature. *Women and Birth, 28*, 1, 40–46.

Rosswood, E. (2016). *Journey to same-sex parenthood: Firsthand advice, tips, and stories from lesbian and gay couples.* Far Hills, NJ: New Horizon Press.

Ryan, A. S., Pratt, W. F., Wysong, J. L., Lewandowski, G., McNally, J. W., & Krieger, F. W. (1991). A comparison of breast-feeding data from the national surveys of family growth and the Ross Laboratories mothers' surveys. *American Journal of Public Health 81*, 8, 1048–1052.

Sadikman, L. (N/D). Don't ask moms if they're breastfeeding. Ask this instead. *Scary Mommy.* Retrieved from https://www.scarymommy.com/dont-ask-breastfeeding/.

Scagell. (May 22, 2018). Mom's have feelings about Target labeling breastfeeding supplies 'Natural Feeding.' *Scary Mommy.* Retrieved from https://www.scarymommy.com/target-natural-feeding-sign-causing-arguments/.

Scary Mommy. (2017). About. Retrieved from https://www.scarymommy.com/about-scary-Mommy/

Scary Mommy, February 21, 2018 [Instagram post]. Retrieved from https://www.instagram.com/p/BfecbJIg1Gm/.

Scary Mommy, May 28, 2018 [Instagram post]. Retrieved from https://www.instagram.com/p/BjVNRYuA5jz/.

Scary Mommy, August 28, 2018 [Instagram post]. Retrieved from https://www.instagram.com/p/BnCvmk1ASCa/.

Scary Mommy, October 15, 2017 [Instagram post]. Retrieved from https://www.instagram.com/p/BaRFxs8FN7e/.

Schneider, G. (2003). *Conservatism in American since 1930: A reader.* New York: University of New York Press.

Sears, W., Sears, M., Sears, R., & Sears, J. (2003). *The baby book: Everything you need to know about your baby from birth to age two.* New York: Little Brown.

Shogun, C. J. (2006). Coolidge and Reagan: The rhetorical influence of Silent Cal on the Great Communicator. *Rhetoric & Public Affairs, 9*, 215–234.

Shome, R. (2011) 'Global motherhood': The transnational intimacies of white femininity. *Critical Studies in Media Communication, 28*, 388–406. doi: 10.1080/15295036.2011.589861

Shoshana, A. (2014). Discursive alliances and clashes in everyday life. *Sociological Spectrum*, 34, 99–113. doi: 10.1080/02732173.2014.877308

Shuman, A. J. (2003). A concise history of infant formula (twists and turns included). *Contemporary Pediatrics, 91*, 2, 91–103.

Smith, C. (2017). Ronald Reagan's rhetorical re-invention of conservatism. *Quarterly Journal of Speech, 103*, 33–65.

Smokler, J. (N/D). Jill Smokler is a noted entrepreneur, social influencer, New York Times bestselling author, and community builder. *JillSmokler.com.* Retrieved from https://jillsmokler.com.

Solomon, M. (1979). The 'Positive Woman's' journey: A mythical analysis of the rhetoric of the STOP ERA. *The Quarterly Journal of Speech, 65*, 262–274.

Sometimes Kids are Dicks, November 11, 2017 [Instagram post]. Retrieved from https://www.instagram.com/p/BnH9woYBpc_/.

Sometimes Kids are Dicks, November 11, 2017 [Instagram post]. Retrieved from https://www.instagram.com/p/BbWxJglj3MT/.

Sometimes Kids are Dicks, July 26, 2018 [Instagram post]. Retrieved from https://www.instagram.com/p/Blt2adtBtkM/.

Sometimes Kids are Dicks, July 26, 2018 [Instagram post]. Retrieved from https://www.instagram.com/p/Bm4eEK0hcm7/.

Sometimes Kids are Dicks, August 24, 2018 [Instagram post]. Retrieved from https://www.instagram.com/p/Bm3vAgYhY8U/.

Sometimes Kids are Dicks, August 24, 2018 [Instagram post]. Retrieved from https://www.instagram.com/p/Bm4eEK0hcm7/.

Sometimes Kids are Dicks, August 31, 2018 [Instagram post]. Retrieved from https://www.instagram.com/p/BnKE_JihCSg/.

Swanson, K. (August 27, 2013). *Black breastfeeding week: Interview with cofounder Anayah Sangodele-Ayoka*. Retrieved on September 17, 2018 from http://theleakyboob.com/tag/women-of-color-and-breastfeeding/.

The baby-friendly hospital initiative (N/D). Retrieved December 20, 2018 from https://www.babyfriendlyusa.org/about/.

The Official Site of Pat Robertson. Biography. Retrieved from http://www.patrobertson.com/Biography/index.asp.

The Pregnancy Discrimination Act, 42 US Code Chapter 21 Sec. 701 (k) of Civil Rights Act of 1964 Title VII. Retrieved from https://www.eeoc.gov/laws/statutes/pregnancy.cfm.

The Surgeon General's call to action to support breastfeeding (2011). Washington, DC: U.S. Department of Health and Human Services. Office of the Surgeon General.

Thomas, C. (2007). The baby and the bath water: Disabled women and motherhood in a social context. In A. O'Reilly (Ed.), *Maternal theory: Essential Readings* (pp. 500–519). Bradford, Canada: Demeter Press.

Thulier, D. (2009). Breastfeeding in America: A history of influencing factors. *Journal of Human Lactation*, *25*(1), 85–94. https://doi.org/10.1177/0890334408324452

Travis, C. (1993). *Mismeasure of woman*. Touchtone.

U.S. Census Bureau, Current population survey (2010). Retrieved from http://www.census.gov/prod/2010pubs/p60-238.pdf.

U.S. Department of Health and Human Services. (2011). *The Surgeon General's call to action to support breastfeeding*. Washington, DC: U.S. Department of Health and Human Services. Office of the Surgeon General.

United States Department of Agriculture. (October 17, 2018). Women, Infants, and Children (WIC). *Breastfeeding is a priority in the WIC program*. Retrieved December 11, 2018 from https://www.fns.usda.gov/wic/breastfeeding-priority-wic-program.

United States Department of Health and Human Services. (1979). *Healthy people 1990, Section 3, Chapter 3: Healthy infants*. Washington, DC: Department of Health and Human Services, Public Health Service, Office of the Assistant Secretary of Health: pp. 1–27. Retrieved from http://profiles.nlm.nih.gov/ps/access/NNBBGV.pdf.

United States. Department of Labor. Office of the Solicitor. (1963). Legislative history of the Equal Pay Act of 1963, amending section 6 of the Fair Labor Standards Act of 1938, as amended, Public Law 88-38, 88th Congress, H.R. 6060 and S. 1409. Washington, U.S. G.P.O.

Vandervort, B. (May 21, 1981). U.S., almost alone, casts ballot against code on baby formula. Retrieved from https://www.washingtonpost.com/archive/politics/1981/05/21/us-almost-alone-casts-ballot-against-code-on-baby-formula/818c3212-6a5c-46ea-93ea-617d6291f21b/?noredirect=on&utm_term=.72405e744871.

Wick, M. (2018). *The Mayo Clinic's guide to a healthy pregnancy; revised edition*. Mayo Clinic.

Willetts, M. (N/D). 'Fed is best': One mom's amazing response to the stranger who shamed her for buying baby formula. Parents.com. Retrieved from https://www.parents.com/baby/all-about-babies/fed-is-best-one-moms-amazing-response-to-the-stranger-who-shamed-her-for/.

Williams, V. (March 26, 2016). Adele on breastfeeding: 'The pressure on us is f@*#ing ridiculous,' *Scary Mommy*. Retrieved from https://www.scarymommy.com/adele-rantbreastfeeding-pressure-london-concert/.

Wolf, J. B. (2011). *Is breast best? Taking on the breastfeeding experts and the new high stakes of motherhood*. New York: New York University Press.

Wolf, J. B. (2013). The politics of dissent. *Journal of Women, Politics, & Policy, 34*, 306–316. doi: 10.1080/154477X.2013.835646

Wolfe, M. (June 30, 2015). This day in history: National Organization for Women was founded. The White House Blog. Retrieved from https://obamawhitehouse.archives.gov/blog/2015/06/30/day-history-national-organization-women-was-founded.

Woltersdor, V. (2011). Paradoxes of Precarious Sexualities. *Cultural Studies, 25*, 164–182.

Women in Labor History Timeline. Retrieved from https://www.afscme.org/formembers/womens-leadership-training/leadershiptools/body/Women_in_Labor_History_Timeline.pdf.

Wright, A. L., & Schanler, R. J. (2001). The resurgence of breastfeeding at the end of the second millennium. *The Journal of Nutrition, 131*, 421S–425S.

Wright, T. (N/D). Breastfeeding does not equal success in motherhood. *Scary Mommy*. Retrieved from https://www.scarymommy.com/bottle-feeding-formula-is-not-failure/.

Yeo, E. J. (2005). Constructing and contesting motherhood, 1750–1950. *Hecate, 31*, 2, 4–20.

Zoll, R. (May 15, 2007). Fallwell changed U.S. politics. *The Washington Post*. Retrieved from http://www.washingtonpost.com/wpdyn/content/article/2007/05/15/AR2007051501603.html?noredirect=on.

Index

About the Authors

Loreen N. Olson (PhD, University of Nebraska, Lincoln) conducts research on gender, family, and relational communication, focusing on the dark side of communication and the communicative management of identities on the margins. She has published on the dark side of family communication, intimate partner violence, intimate partner violence related traumatic brain injury, the discourse of motherhood, family secrets, verbal aggressiveness, and the luring communication of child sexual predators. She is the co-author of *The Dark Side of Family Communication* and co-editor of *The Darker Side of Family Communication: The Harmful, the Morally Suspect, and the Socially Inappropriate*. Dr. Olson is a past editor of the *Journal of Family Communication* and a past chair of the Family Communication Division of the National Communication Association.

Jenni M. Simon (PhD, University of Denver) researches gender and cultural issues, as well as the critical and rhetorical intersections that exist between culture and social movements. Her most recent work explores feminism and social change, resistance to women's movements, women in organizations and politics, and the changing role of motherhood in the post-modern area. Dr. Simon has published in *Communication Review, Southern States Communication Journal, Western Communication Journal, Women and Language* and in the *Proceedings on the International Conference of Gender Research*. She is the co-editor *of Michelle Obama: First Lady, American Rhetor* and the author of *Consuming Desire and Agency: Stories of Love, Laughter, and Empowerment*. Dr. Simon is a past chair of the Southern States Communication Association's Gender and Women's Studies Division. She is the current editor of the *Carolinas Communication Associations' Annual.*

Lightning Source UK Ltd.
Milton Keynes UK
UKHW040952080120
356571UK00002B/215/P

9 781498 531290